CancerTips

A Handbook for Cancer Prevention
and Management

# CancerTips

## A Handbook for Cancer Prevention and Management

**JAMES M. METZ, M.D.**
Assistant Professor
Department of Radiation Oncology
Editor-in-Chief, OncoLink
University of Pennsylvania Medical Center
Hospital of the University of Pennsylvania
Philadelphia, Pennsylvania

LIPPINCOTT WILLIAMS & WILKINS
A **Wolters Kluwer** Company
Philadelphia • Baltimore • New York • London
Buenos Aires • Hong Kong • Sydney • Tokyo

*Acquisitions Editor:* Jonathan W. Pine, Jr.
*Developmental Editor:* Joyce A. Murphy
*Production Editor:* Melanie Bennitt
*Manufacturing Manager:* Colin Warnock
*Cover Designer:* Karen Quigley
*Compositor:* Maryland Composition
*Printer:* Vicks Lithograph & Printing

© 2002 by LIPPINCOTT WILLIAMS & WILKINS
530 Walnut Street
Philadelphia, PA 19106 USA
LWW.com

Printed in the USA

Library of Congress Cataloging-in-Publication Data

CancerTips : a handbook for cancer prevention and management / edited by James M. Metz.
   p. ; cm.
 Includes index.
 ISBN 0-7817-2564-X
  1. Cancer—Handbooks, Manuals, etc. 2. Cancer—Popular works.
  I. Metz, James M.
 [DNLM: 1. Neoplasms—prevention & control—Handbooks.
 2. Neoplasms—prevention & control—Resource Guides.
 3. Alternative Medicine—Handbooks. 4. Alternative Medicine—
 Resource Guides. QZ 39 C2163 2000]
 RC262.5 .C36 2000
 616.99'4—dc21

                                                                    2001042532

Care has been taken to confirm the accuracy of the information presented and to describe generally accepted practices. However, the author and publisher are not responsible for errors or omissions or for any consequences from application of the information in this book and make no warranty, expressed or implied, with respect to the currency, completeness, or accuracy of the contents of the publication. Application of this information in a particular situation remains the professional responsibility of the practitioner.

The author and publisher have exerted every effort to ensure that drug selection and dosage set forth in this text are in accordance with current recommendations and practice at the time of publication. However, in view of ongoing research, changes in government regulations, and the constant flow of information relating to drug therapy and drug reactions, the reader is urged to check the package insert for each drug for any change in indications and dosage and for added warnings and precautions. This is particularly important when the recommended agent is a new or infrequently employed drug.

Some drugs and medical devices presented in this publication have Food and Drug Administration (FDA) clearance for limited use in restricted research settings. It is the responsibility of the health care provider to ascertain the FDA status of each drug or device planned for use in their clinical practice.

                                        10 9 8 7 6 5 4 3 2 1

# CONTENTS

## I. CANCER PREVENTION AND SCREENING

## II. DEALING WITH THE SIDE EFFECTS OF CANCER TREATMENT

## III.   SEXUALITY ISSUES

## IV.   PHYSICIAN AND PATIENT INTERACTIONS

## V.   ONCOLOGIC EMERGENCIES

## VI.   ALTERNATIVE MEDICINE

## VII. MISCELLANEOUS TOPICS

## VIII. INTERNET GUIDE TO USEFUL CANCER INFORMATION

## IX. CANCER WORKBOOK

# PREFACE

*CancerTips* has arisen from a desire to provide clear, concise information that can always remain at a cancer patient's fingertips. I first began writing *CancerTips* two years ago when I joined the OncoLink staff. They have rapidly become the most popular documents on the OncoLink website. The tips are summaries of the most important information that a cancer patient needs to know. They are not meant to include every detail, only the most important points.

This book is designed to be carried in a purse or even a pocket. Take it with you to your physician's appointments. If you have symptoms, look them up in the book and ask your physician if the recommendations are appropriate in your particular case. If you are having specific side effects, ask your doctor about the recommended medications to see if they are right for you. This book will help you to become an active member of your healthcare team. Take charge of your situation. Stay involved.

Section I provides important information on the prevention and screening for cancer. This section will benefit anyone who is interested in cancer prevention and early detection of cancer. Recommendations on screening patients with a previous cancer are also included. Section II addresses some of the most common side effects of cancer treatments. Recommendations are made to help patients minimize these side effects and treat them once they occur. Sexuality and cancer, physician/patient interactions, and oncologic emergencies are discussed in the subsequent sections. Many of the most popular alternative medical practices are discussed in Section VI. Specifically, the available scientific background, safety, cost, and current recommendations regarding the use of these treatments in the cancer patient are included. An Internet guide to useful cancer sites is also included.

One of the most useful sections in this book may be the Workbook. This will help you keep important information about physicians, medications, appointments, and treatments in one place. These charts are designed to facilitate visits with your physicians. Using these charts will help you present information in a clear and concise format. The pages can be photocopied and added to your medical chart. This allows you to spend more time discussing issues that are important to you instead of fumbling for information.

This book has been an ambitious project and I hope it will find a valued place in the lives of many cancer patients.

*James M. Metz, M.D.*

# FOREWORD

The ability to distribute cancer information over the Internet has revolutionized our approach to patient education. It is equally noteworthy that we can simultaneously broadcast this information worldwide to assist patients and, in doing so, their professional caretakers. The paradigm shift in publishing is undeniably as significant as the development of the printing press. OncoLink, the source from which such information has emanated, represents among the best that cancer professionals have to offer to their patients en mass. Yet, it is no more than a tool and vehicle that is only as good and useful as the content it seeks to provide.

When Dr. Metz came to us with the idea of creating tips for cancer patients on OncoLink, we were immediately intrigued. We recognized this project as an extraordinary milestone in our goal to help educate and care for those confronting cancer.

Now we have reached an impasse. OncoTips are among the most popular postings accessed on OncoLink. Millions have seen, read, and followed them. Unfortunately, this represents only a fraction of those confronting cancer on a daily basis and benefiting from the information. By providing these tips in the format of a book, and including a workbook that patients can use to record helpful treatment information, we believe we can take this project a step further. Not only will we be able to reach out to many more users, but we will also provide them with a handbook that we hope will be invaluable as they course through therapy. Finally, all proceeds that we receive will be used towards OncoLink to further our mission.

We sincerely hope you find this book informative and useful. We welcome you to visit OncoLink to find additional information about cancer and cancer treatment. New tips are being posted regularly, and some may even be incorporated into future versions of this handbook.

It is our sincere hope that such resources become unnecessary in the coming decades. Until such time, we remain committed to being the most reputable sources of cancer information for patients and professionals. *CancerTips* from OncoLink is but one step in the process of eliminating this disease and its consequences.

*Joel W. Goldwein, M.D.*
*Founder, OncoLink*

# CANCER PREVENTION AND SCREENING

*CancerTip*          **Reasons to Quit Smoking**

## INCREASED RISK OF LUNG CANCER IS NOT THE ONLY REASON TO QUIT SMOKING

The Great American Smokeout, which is promoted by the American Cancer Society, is scheduled in mid-November each year. It is hoped that millions will quit smoking for a day and possibly for life. It is well known that smoking causes lung cancer. In 2001, it is expected 169,500 Americans will be diagnosed with lung cancer. Unfortunately, most of these people will die of their disease.

There are a number of other diseases that smoking has been associated with over the years. Many of these diseases have high mortality rates. If lung cancer is not reason enough to quit smoking, maybe some of the other diseases associated with smoking will encourage people to quit the habit.

There are a number of other cancers related to smoking. Cancer of the head and neck region, particularly cancer of the voice box and mouth, are strongly associated with smoking. Esophageal cancer is also caused by smoking. It has recently been shown that smoking increases the risk of developing leukemia. Other organs with increased incidence of cancer in smokers include the stomach, kidney, bladder, and pancreas. Female smokers have an increased risk of developing cervical cancer.

There are many other diseases besides cancer that are related to smoking. Heart disease, the number one killer in America, has a much higher incidence in smokers. Debilitating lung diseases such as emphysema and chronic bronchitis are almost only seen in smokers. The blood vessels in the arms and legs can become narrowed, causing cramping and weakness in heavy smokers. There is also a much higher risk of strokes in smokers.

Male smokers have a higher incidence of impotence owing to circulation problems in the pelvic area. They tend to develop potency problems at a much younger age compared with non-smokers. Unfortunately, impotence from this cause is not as responsive to many of the new impotency treatments. The longer a man smokes, the higher the risk.

Female smokers may also have significant problems with arousal and sexual stimulation. Pregnant smokers have a higher incidence of low-birth-weight babies and increased risk of infant mortality. Female smokers also have more complications related to the use of birth control pills than nonsmokers.

It is important that those smokers who have developed cancer quit smoking. Those who are cured of their cancer are at much higher risk of developing a second malignancy if they continue to use tobacco. It is also much more difficult to tolerate treatments for cancer while smoking. There is increased incidence of certain side effects of conventional cancer treatments with the interaction of tobacco smoke.

If you are not worried about yourself, you should also consider the health of others. Family, friends, and coworkers are at risk to develop some of the above-mentioned diseases from exposure to second hand smoke. Children are also at risk of developing reactive airway diseases. Infants are at increased risk of experiencing fluid in the middle ear and other lung disorders including pneumonia and bronchitis.

OncoLink strongly encourages its users to participate in the Great American Smokeout. If you are not a smoker, encourage the smokers around you to try and quit for a day. For more information on the Great American Smokeout, visit the Great American Smokeout website sponsored by the American Cancer Society (http://www2.cancer.org/gas/).

*CancerTip*

# Colorectal Cancer Screening

It is estimated that more than 135,400 Americans will develop colon cancer or rectal cancer in 2001. It is the second most common cause of death from cancer in the United States. Colorectal cancer can be treated most effectively when it is discovered at an early stage of disease.

There are a number of risk factors associated with the development of colorectal cancer. Hereditary colon polyps, cancer family syndromes, and a history of colorectal cancer in a parent or sibling place the individual at a higher risk. A personal history of benign colon polyps, previous colorectal cancer, or inflammatory bowel disease places the individual at higher risk. However, less than one third of patients diagnosed with colorectal cancer have high-risk features. There is an increased risk of developing colorectal cancer with increasing age. For this reason, it is recommended that all individuals over the age of 50 participate in colorectal cancer screening.

There are a number of screening tests used to detect colorectal cancer:

## DIGITAL RECTAL EXAMINATION

The physician inserts a gloved finger into the rectum and feels for any abnormalities. If no blood is visible on the gloved finger, fecal occult blood testing is performed (see later). To date, there has not been significant evidence that the rectal examination has had any effect on mortality when used alone as a screening test. It should be used in combination with the tests noted in the following sections.

## FECAL OCCULT BLOOD TESTING

Special cards are utilized to test for occult blood (blood not seen by the naked eye). Patients can place a small sample of feces on the card at home, or the physician can place a sample on the card after a digital rectal examination. A special chemical is used by a laboratory to determine if blood is present. It should be noted that many things could cause a positive occult blood test. If you have a positive test, further studies are needed. Fecal occult blood testing on a yearly basis for an individual 45 to 80 years of age has been shown to decrease mortality from colorectal cancer.

## SIGMOIDOSCOPY

A sigmoidoscope is a thin tube with a light at the end, which is placed into the rectum. It can evaluate the distal colon and the rectum for polyps, tumors, and other abnormalities. Regular screening in individuals older than 50 years of age may decrease mortality from colorectal cancer. There has been notable debate over the best screening interval. You should discuss this issue with your physician.

## COLONOSCOPY

The colonoscope is much longer than a sigmoidoscope, so that the entire colon can be viewed. Patients are usually sedated for a colonoscopy procedure. A colonoscopy may be recommended for patients who are at high risk for colorectal cancer, have abnormalities on a sigmoidoscopy, or have unexplained fecal occult blood.

## BARIUM ENEMA

A barium enema is an x-ray study of the colon and rectum. Barium is contrast material that is given by enema before taking x-ray studies. This procedure allows the colon and rectum to be visualized and abnormalities can be evaluated. The patient is placed on a table that moves so the barium can be followed as it moves through the bowel.

The American Cancer Society recommends three courses of action beginning at the age of 50 years. The patient and physician can choose the best screening method for their circumstances. These include:

- Annual fecal occult blood tests, together with a flexible sigmoidoscopy and digital rectal examination every 5 years.

OR

- Colonoscopy with digital rectal examination every 10 years

OR

- Double contrast barium enema with digital rectal examination every 5 to 10 years

*CancerTip*         **Mammography**

Owing to the introduction of mammography, breast cancers are being diagnosed at an earlier stage of disease. There has also been a marked increase in the incidence of ductal carcinoma *in situ* (DCIS) of the breast that has corresponded to the increased use of mammography. When breast cancer is diagnosed at an earlier stage, there is a better chance of cure and long-term survival. Breast-conserving therapies can be used when the breast cancer is detected early.

There are different types of mammograms that are performed. The screening mammogram is a two-view examination of each breast. It is only used to screen asymptomatic patients. It is not used for patients who have a suspicious mass on physical examination. The diagnostic mammogram is performed to define further, the location of an abnormality detected during a screening mammogram or to clarify an indeterminate lesion. It is also performed in patients who have a suspicious lesion on physical examination or patients who have had breast cancer in the past and were treated with breast-conservation techniques. Patients who have had breast augmentation also require diagnostic mammograms with specialized views of the breast. Specialized techniques and magnified spot views are used in the diagnostic mammogram.

The radiologist looks for specific mammographic findings considered suspicious for malignancy. The radiologist also looks for any new changes in the breasts when compared with previous mammograms. It is important that the patient has mammograms performed at the same institution each time or brings mammograms that were previously performed for comparison purposes.

There have been eight large randomized clinical trials performed to evaluate the utility of mammograms. Evidence sug-
gests a powerful impact of mammography for women 50 to 69
years. No trial has yet recorded convincing evidence of a reduction in mortality rate for women aged 40 to 49 years of age.
There have not been enough women older than 70 years of age
included in these trials to make definitive recommendations
for that age group. Major health organizations have each reviewed the available data regarding mammography and made
different conclusions. The most controversial age group is
among patients who are 40 to 49 years old.

The current American Cancer Society Screening Recommendations are as follows:

- Mammograms every 1 to 2 years for women in their 40s
- Mammograms yearly for patients 50 years and older

One must remember that the mammogram is only one of
the tools used for screening breast cancer patients. There is no
mammographic abnormality in 15% of the patients diagnosed
with cancer. Monthly breast self-examination and regular
physical examinations by your physician continue to be
extremely important in the early diagnosis of breast cancer.

*CancerTip*        **Breast Self-Examination**

An estimated 193,700 women will develop breast cancer in 2001. Clearly, those women who are diagnosed with cancer at an early stage of disease have a better chance of cure. Important screening techniques include breast self-examination, breast examinations by trained healthcare providers, and mammography. Some breast cancers never show up on a mammogram, so it is important to perform breast self-examinations.

The American Cancer Society recommends that women 20 years of age and older practice monthly breast self-examination. Those children and adolescent's who received radiation therapy to the chest region for cancer such as Hodgkin's disease should be taught the technique at an even earlier age. Breasts should be examined once each month, 7 to 10 days after the start of the menstrual period. The texture and contour of the breast change in relation to the menstrual cycle. Postmenopausal women should pick the same date each month (e.g., the first day of the month, mortgage due date).

There are two major parts to the breast self-examination: visual inspection and palpation. Visual inspection consists of standing in front of a mirror with the breasts uncovered. Observe the contour of each breast. Notice the size of each breast, shape, and nipple position. Make mental notes of each of these parameters and compare for any changes each month. Next, raise arms over your head and note any changes in the skin or dimpling of the skin. Then place your hands on your hips and squeeze your chest muscles while looking for dimpling or skin changes.

Palpation consists of feeling the breasts with the pads of your three longest fingers of one hand. First, while standing, cradle the left breast with the left hand. Gently feel the breast with the three longest fingers on the right hand. Note any lumps or bumps. Note any changes from the last exam. Next, cradle the right breast with the right hand and palpate with the left hand. Again note any lumps or changes.

After you have palpated the breasts while standing, lie down on your back with the left arm behind the head. Palpate the entire breast with the three longest fingers on the right hand. There are various techniques that can be used so that all of the breast tissue is palpated:

a) Start at the areola (pigmented area surrounding the nipple) and go around the breast clockwise in progressively larger circles until the entire breast has been felt.

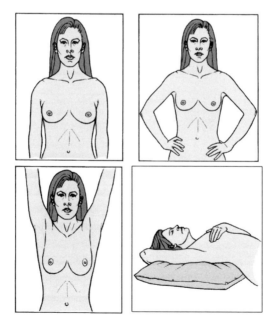

b) Divide the breast into equal wedges like a pie and examine each wedge from the nipple out to the edge. Then repeat from the outside to the areola.

c) Use overlapping vertical or horizontal strips to cover all of the breast tissue.

With each of these techniques, make sure to palpate the area beneath the collar bone and the armpit. Now repeat the procedure on the right breast by placing the right arm behind the head and palpating with the three longest fingers on the left hand.

Do not hesitate to ask your physician about the proper technique for breast self-examination. It may take several times until you feel comfortable with the technique and note the normal texture and consistency of your breast tissue. If you find a lump, feel unusual tenderness or pain, notice changes in the color of the skin, or find secretion from a nipple, notify your physician. These symptoms do not mean you have cancer. Many other conditions can cause these changes. Make an appointment with your healthcare provider for a formal evaluation. It is important to follow up on any changes or unusual symptoms related to your breast self-examination.

*CancerTip*        **Pap Smear**

There has been a dramatic decrease in the death rate from cervical cancer since the introduction of the Pap smear by Dr. Papaniculaou in the1940s. It rapidly became the most effective screening test for cancer ever introduced. The Pap smear can detect both precancerous changes and cancer of the cervix. By detecting lesions that are precancerous, specific treatments can be used to prevent a woman from developing cervical cancer. It is estimated there will be 4,400 deaths due to cervical cancer in 2001.

   Pap smears are performed along with a pelvic examination by a physician or other specially trained healthcare professionals. A speculum is inserted into the vagina so that the cervix can be visualized. For those patients who have had a hysterectomy with removal of the cervix, the vaginal cuff is visually inspected. For those patients with an intact cervix, a sample of cells is taken from the outer portion of the cervix using a wooden or plastic spatula. A small brush is then used to take a second sample from the inner part of the cervix. Both of these samples are immediately placed on glass slides and preserved with a special spray. For those patients without a cervix, a sample is taken from the vaginal cuff. Following the Pap smear, a pelvic examination is performed.

   The American Cancer Society recommends that all women begin yearly Pap smears and pelvic examinations at the age of 18 or when they become sexually active, whichever comes first. It is recommended women continue with pelvic exams annually. Pap smears should be performed annually for at least three consecutive negative Pap smears in a row. The test may be performed less often at the discretion of the healthcare provider after three annual normal Pap smears.

For those patients who have been treated for a cervical or endometrial cancer, more frequent Pap smears are recommended. Typically, pelvic examiantions and Pap smears are performed every 3 to 6 months in the first few years after completion of treatment with surgery or radiation therapy. The highest chance for recurrence of cancer is in the first 3 years, so careful follow-up is recommended.

*CancerTip*        **CA-125 Tumor Marker**

CA-125 is a blood test that is typically used in the management of patients with ovarian cancer. The CA-125 level can be elevated above the normal level in a variety of other conditions besides ovarian cancer. Because most patients with ovarian cancer have an elevated CA-125 level, it is a good test to use to follow the patient's response to a particular treatment (the value decreases if a treatment is working or increases if the tumor is growing).

It was hoped that the CA-125 blood test could also be applied as a screening test to detect ovarian cancer at an early stage in women. A good screening test needs to be safe, specific, and make a difference in survival due to early initiation of treatment. A number of studies with many thousands of patients have not shown a benefit to using CA-125 as a screening test for the following reasons:

- A number of common benign conditions cause an increase in CA-125 including normal menses, pregnancy, fibroids, endometriosis, and pelvic inflammatory disease
- Nongynecologic conditions that elevate the CA-125 level include pancreatitis (inflammation of the pancreas), liver cirrhosis, recent abdominal surgery, and radiation therapy treatments
- Other malignant tumors such as breast, lung, colon, and pancreas can increase the CA-125

Because so many other conditions can elevate the CA-125 level, this test has a significant number of false-positive results. If every patient with a positive result underwent additional work-up, many patients would require a surgical exploration of the abdomen to rule out definitively a diagnosis of ovarian cancer. Surgery can cause significant side effects and, even rarely, death. It also turns out that studies have shown no impact on the rate of death by using the CA-125 as a screening test. Thus, as a screening test in a patient without a diagnosis of ovarian cancer or strong suspicion of its presence, CA-125 does not fulfill the important requirements of a screening test. The risks do not outweigh the benefits, the test is not very specific in its diagnosis, and it has not been shown to impact survival significantly.

Routine screening of asymptomatic patients with a CA-125 level is not recommended. However, there are individual instances in which getting a CA-125 test is prudent. Some physicians still favor the test in patients with a strong family history of ovarian cancer and combine screening for ovarian cancer with pelvic and ultrasound examinations. It is clearly indicated to have regular CA-125 blood tests that patients who were previously diagnosed with ovarian cancer to follow response of treatment or catch a recurrence at an early stage.

# Prostate Specific Antigen (PSA)

Prostate cancer is the most common cancer diagnosis in men. According to the American Cancer Society, approximately 198,100 men will be diagnosed with prostate cancer in 2001. Screening for prostate cancer has gained increased importance with the development of the prostate specific antigen (PSA) blood test. Many patients do not have a palpable abnormality on the digital rectal examination (DRE), and an elevated PSA is the first sign of prostate cancer.

The screening PSA test is the most common type of PSA test used in the United States. It has an upper limit of normal of 4.0 nanograms per milliliter (ng/mL) in serum. This is based on a 50-year-old man. There can be adjustments in the normal level based on the age of the patient. Benign conditions such as benign prostatic hypertrophy (BPH) and inflammation of the prostate (prostatitis) may cause elevations of PSA. Cancer of the prostate gland can also cause a rise in the PSA blood test. PSA values in the 4 to 10 ng/mL range are considered borderline high, and the condition may be evaluated with special types of PSA tests. Values of greater than 10 ng/mL or any patient with an abnormal digital rectal examination should have a biopsy of the prostate to rule out the presence of prostate cancer. It must be remembered that there is great variability in the presentation of prostate cancer and these values are not absolute.

There are a number of specialized PSA tests that are used to help differentiate between elevated PSA due to benign conditions and those elevations due to prostate cancer. These include the free PSA, PSA velocity, and PSA density tests. These tests can be further discussed with your physician if your PSA is in the borderline high range on a screening PSA test.

The PSA test must be evaluated in conjunction with the patient's history, physical examination, and radiologic studies (e.g., ultrasound examinations). PSA is one tool in the screening of prostate cancer. It is clear that patients are now diagnosed at an earlier stage of disease than before the introduction of PSA. Prostate cancer has more options for treatment and better chance of cure when diagnosed at an earlier stage of disease. OncoLink strongly supports the current American Cancer Society recommendations for prostate cancer screening:

- Annual PSA and DRE for men 50 years and older
- Annual PSA and DRE for younger men who are of African descent or men with two or more first-degree relatives (father or brothers) affected by prostate cancer

*CancerTip*

# Screening for Testicular Cancer

It is estimated that there will be 7,200 cases of testicular cancer in 2001 in the United States. It is the most common cancer in men between 15 and 34 years of age. This is an age when many individuals feel "invincible"; thus, it is more difficult to get patients to practice screening on a regular basis. Although most patients can be cured of testicular cancer, it is estimated that 400 American men will die of this disease in 2001.

Most testicular cancers present with a mass in the scrotum that can be felt by the man. Sometimes patients complain of a dull ache in the groin, abdomen, or testicle. Fortunately, testicular cancer is a highly curable disease, which makes screening very important. It is always better to catch cancer at an early stage of disease to obtain the best outcome.

Testicular self-examination is as important to men as breast self-examination is to women. Testicular self-examination should be performed on a monthly basis as recommended by the American Cancer Society. It is best performed after a warm shower because this is when the testes are most descended and the scrotal skin is relaxed. This will allow for a more complete examination. Roll each testicle between the thumb and fingers. Feel for any lumps or nodules. You may feel the epididymis, which is a soft structure on the top of the testicle that is involved in sperm storage and transport. If any abnormalities are felt, notify your physician so that a formal examination can be performed.

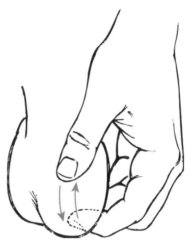

*CancerTip*        **Sun Protection**

The most common cancer diagnosed in the United States is skin cancer. In 2001, there will be over one million new cases of skin cancer diagnosed. The most common types of skin cancer include basal cell carcinoma and squamous cell carcinoma. Melanoma will account for approximately 51,400 new cases of skin cancer in 2001.

Basal cell carcinomas occur on skin that has had significant exposure to sunlight. It is typically treated with surgery. Radiation therapy may be used when surgery will cause disfigurement or there are high-risk features that make it likely to recur. There is a very low risk for spread to lymph nodes or distant sites in the body.

Squamous cell carcinomas of the skin also occur on sun exposed areas of the body. They are treated similarly to basal cell carcinomas. However, there is a slightly higher risk of spread to lymph nodes and distant sites. Both basal and squamous cell carcinomas are typically cured with local treatment when the disease is caught early.

Melanoma is a much more aggressive type of skin cancer. It can even occur on areas of the body not exposed to ultraviolet light. It has a significantly higher risk of spread to lymph nodes and distant sites within the body. It is treated with much more aggressive surgery and sometimes lymph node removal. Patients with advanced lesions may also receive chemotherapy and radiation therapy. The earlier the lesion is detected, the higher the cure rate.

The best way to avoid skin cancer is to protect oneself and loved ones from the rays of the sun. It is important to take precautions during every season of the year, not just summer. The following tips may help reduce your risk of developing skin cancer:

- Avoid exposure to the sun during the peak hours of 11 AM to 3 PM.
- Wear protective clothing during peak times of the day. Clothes should be tight weaves. Cotton T-shirts are only equivalent to a SPF-6 lotion.
- Wear a wide brim hat to protect your head and face.
- Avoid tanning salons. The ultraviolet light from the tanning booths can cause skin cancer and make the skin age prematurely.
- Generously apply broad-spectrum sunscreen with a high SPF. Use those sunscreens that are water resistant if you plan to swim or exercise.
- Use sun protection on cloudy days because ultraviolet light passes through clouds.
- Avoid any sun exposure if you are taking medications that increase your sun sensitivity.
- Make sure to wear sun protection while skiing. Snow reflects the light and the intensity of the suns rays increases at high altitudes.
- Always have new skin lesions checked by a physician promptly.

# Early Detection of Melanoma

There will be an estimated 51,400 new cases of melanoma diagnosed in 2001. Melanoma is highly curable when detected at an early stage of disease. Unfortunately, many patients present with advanced disease and ultimately the treatment fails. Early detection of melanoma requires regular self-examination of the skin. Professional examination by a physician should also be performed on a yearly basis.

The mnemonic "ABCDE" has been developed to help people recognize melanoma at an early stage. When performing self-examination of the skin, think of the mnemonic to help you recognize any suspicious lesions.

A = Asymmetry—the growth is not perfectly round. It has an irregular shape.

B = Border—the border of the lesion is not smooth and regular.

C = Color—any skin growth that is more than one color should be evaluated. Benign moles usually are one color.

D = Diameter—any growth larger than 5 mL (1/4 inch) should be evaluated.

E = Elevation—any lesion that is elevated or develops a bump should be brought to your physician's attention.

The entire skin surface needs to be evaluated. This procedure requires the use of a mirror and multiple positions to evaluate the back, skin folds, and creases. Always report new growths or changes in moles or skin marks to your physician for formal evaluation.

# DEALING WITH THE SIDE EFFECTS OF CANCER TREATMENT

# Diarrhea

Diarrhea is a common side effect of chemotherapy and radiation therapy. Chemotherapy drugs affect the lining of the intestinal tract. Radiation therapy causes diarrhea when the area treated includes the abdomen and pelvis. Radiation seed implants for prostate cancer can also cause diarrhea. Fortunately, this is a temporary side effect in the vast majority of patients. Diarrhea can be effectively managed in most patients who follow these recommendations:

- Start with clear fluids, broth, and toast.
- Slowly add foods back into your diet as tolerated.
- Rice, bananas, apple sauce, and toast are usually well tolerated.
- Eat small, frequent meals. Do not eat large meals.
- Eat foods at room temperature.
- Avoid milk products, including cheese and ice cream.
- Avoid fresh fruits.
- Cook all vegetable well. Raw vegetables are difficult to digest.
- Avoid greasy, fatty, spicy, or fried foods.
- Refrain from taking fiber supplements such as Metamucil or calcium polycarbophil (FiberCon).
- Drink plenty of water (at least eight glasses a day) because there is a risk of becoming dehydrated.
- As the diarrhea improves, add more foods such as pasta, potatoes, and meats to your diet.
- If the diarrhea lasts more than 24 hours, notify your physician.

- You should consult your physician before taking any over-the-counter antidiarrhea medications such as loperamide (Imodium) or attapulgite (Kaopectate). These medications can be very effective, but they may not be appropriate in your particular situation.

*CancerTip*            # Dry Mouth (Xerostomia)

Dry mouth is most commonly caused by radiation therapy directed at the head and neck region of the body. Radiation may irreversibly affect the production and quality of saliva in the major and minor salivary glands. A number of medications may also induce xerostomia. Dry mouth may affect the patient's speech, taste sensation, ability to swallow, and the use of dentures. Many patients complain of a sore or burning sensation, cracked lips, and cuts in the corners of the mouth. There is also an increased risk of cavities and periodontal disease owing to the fact that there is less saliva available to cleanse the teeth and gums.

Currently there are clinical trials investigating radioprotectors, which are given at the time of radiation therapy in an attempt to prevent xerostomia. If you are going to receive radiation therapy to the head and neck region you may wish to discuss these clinical trials with your radiation oncologist. If you have developed xerostomia, there are management strategies that can effectively deal with your dry mouth and prevent cavities and periodontal disease. Try to follow these simple guidelines:

- Perform oral hygiene at least four times per day (after each meal and before bedtime).
- Your mouth should be rinsed and wiped immediately after meals.
- Dentures need to be brushed and rinsed after meals.
- Only use toothpaste with fluoride when brushing.
- Keep water handy to moisten the mouth.
- Apply prescription strength fluoride gel at bedtime.

- Rinse with salt and baking soda solution four to six times a day (1/2 tsp salt, 1/2 tsp baking soda, and 8 oz of water).
- Avoid liquids and foods with a high sugar content.
- Avoid rinses containing alcohol.
- Use moisturizer regularly on the lips (e.g., Chapstick).
- Salivary substitutes or artificial saliva preparations may relieve discomfort by temporarily wetting the mouth and replacing some of the constituents of saliva.
- Oral pilocarpine (Salagen) is the only drug approved by the Food and Drug Administration (FDA) to stimulate saliva secretion from the remaining salivary glands. It is not a drug for everyone with dry mouth, and it can only be obtained with a prescription from your doctor. Ask your physician if you are a candidate for this medication.

*CancerTip* **Nausea**

Nausea is a common side effect of cancer treatment. It can be stimulated by chemotherapy, radiation therapy, or the cancer itself. Patients typically develop aversions to certain foods and strong aromas frequently trigger nausea. Large amounts of food can make someone anxious and subsequently nauseated. The idea of sitting at a table for a large meal three times a day can become a chore.

Fortunately, nausea can be managed through a combination of medications and behavioral changes. Medications such as ondansetron (Zofran), granisetron (Kytril), prochlorperazine (Compazine), dexamethasone (Decadron), and metoclopramide may be prescribed by your physician to help control nausea. The medication is chosen on an individual basis depending on your situation. Always follow the specific recommendations of your physician on taking these medications because they may cause other side effects.

What you eat, the way you eat, and how you eat may all contribute to nausea. Here are some simple recommendations to help prevent and control nausea:

- Eat small, frequent (five to six) meals, instead of three large meals each day.
- Eat the largest meal at a time of day when you are least nauseated (morning for many people).
- Avoid sweet, spicy, fatty, or fried foods.
- Eat and drink slowly, chew food thoroughly so it is easily digestible.
- Fresh vegetables should be cooked rather than eaten raw.

- Consider shakes or liquid nutritional supplements such as Ensure, Carnation, and Sustacal to help maintain your nutrition.
- Avoid aromas by eating meals cold or at room temperature.
- Enlist friends and family members to cook so you can avoid aromas in the kitchen.
- Eat dry, bland foods such as crackers or toast before meals.
- Rest in a chair after eating, avoid reclining because this may trigger reflux, nausea, and vomiting.
- Aerobic exercise may decrease the nausea associated with chemotherapy.
- Anticipatory nausea associated with chemotherapy is best controlled with relaxation techniques.

If nausea hits:

- Take deep breaths and relax.
- Chew ice chips until nausea has passed.
- Sip small quantities of a clear "flat" soda (such as ginger ale).
- As you feel better, gradually add other foods back into your diet.

# Esophagitis

Esophagitis is an inflammation of the esophagus that causes pain and discomfort with swallowing. The esophagus is a muscular tube that connects the throat to the stomach. Esophagitis is a common side effect of cancer treatment. Radiation therapy and chemotherapy may cause the cancer patient to develop esophagitis.

Radiation therapy may cause esophagitis in patients who are receiving treatment to the chest and neck area. This may include patients with lung cancer, Hodgkin's disease, non-Hodgkin's lymphoma, and head and neck cancers. After two to three weeks of radiation therapy, these patients may begin to notice discomfort with swallowing. Patients typically complain of burning in the neck and chest region. The discomfort usually lasts through the completion of treatment with radiation therapy. The patient will start to notice improvement about 2 weeks after the completion of therapy. In most patients, the esophagitis is resolved 4 to 6 weeks after the radiation therapy has finished.

Chemotherapy may also cause esophagitis. Certain chemotherapy drugs can cause severe irritation of the mucous membranes (mucositis). The esophagus is lined by a mucous membrane and may become irritated. Esophagitis usually occurs days after the administration of chemotherapy instead of weeks like the radiation therapy.

Patients who are on steroid treatments or have a suppressed immune system from their cancer treatments may develop esophagitis due to a fungal infection (esophageal candidiasis). This is generally treated with antifungal oral medications. The esophagitis usually resolves over 1 to 2 weeks of treatment.

There are some ways for a patient to effectively deal with the symptoms of esophagitis:

- Avoid hot or spicy foods.
- Avoid acidic foods such as tomato sauce and orange juice.
- Drink plenty of cool liquids.
- Foods that are cold or at room temperature are easier to tolerate.
- Eat foods that will not distend or stretch the esophagus such as eggs, ice cream, or milk shakes.
- Use nutritional supplements to maintain your weight (e.g., Carnation Instant Breakfast, Ensure, Boost, Scandishake).
- Tell your physician about the symptoms. There are medications that may provide relief of the symptoms.

*CancerTip*               **Fatigue and Cancer**

Fatigue is an overwhelming daily lack of energy, which can have an impact on every aspect of a person's life. It causes the affected individual to feel weak all over and lose interest in those people or activities that they usually enjoy. It is not related to exertion and is not relieved with a good night's sleep. Fatigue may be caused by a number of factors including the diagnosis of cancer, treatments, stress, and other medical conditions.

There are medical causes of fatigue that may be treated effectively. Anemia, which is a low red blood cell count, causes a decrease in the amount of oxygen that is delivered to the body's tissues. There are many causes of anemia, all of which are treated differently. Iron deficiency anemia can be treated with iron supplementation. Slowed production of red blood cells, which can be caused by chemotherapy or chronic illness, can be treated with medications that stimulate the production of red blood cells such as epoetin alfa (Procrit or Epogen). If the red blood cell counts are dangerously low, the patient may require a transfusion.

Hypothyroidism can also cause fatigue. This condition is easily treated with thyroid hormone replacement pills taken once a day. Depression can cause fatigue that can be managed with counseling and medications. Infections, which may also cause fatigue, may be treated with appropriate antibiotics.

A physician should evaluate the patient for any medical causes of fatigue. Fatigue is a common occurrence in the cancer patient. The various cancer treatments and emotional stresses are heavy burdens on the body. The body is waging a war against cancer, and fatigue is a side effect.

Fortunately, there are some simple things that the patient can do to take charge of their life and minimize the effects of fatigue. Here are some recommendations:

- Let your physicians and nurses know that you feel fatigued. Do not hide it. There may be a medical cause that can be easily treated.
- Do not fight fatigue. Rest when you need it. Try to take small naps during the day.
- Try to keep to a regular daily routine that is reasonable.
- Start an exercise program. Exercise can significantly help to relieve fatigue. Start slow at first and work up to a program you can live with.
- Drink lots of water during the day.
- Eat a well-balanced diet with frequent, small meals.
- Avoid caffeine in the evening.
- Take control of the stresses in your life. Take time to put them in perspective.
- Delegate chores. Family and friends are almost always happy to help out in any way they can.

# Hair Loss

Hair loss (alopecia) is a common side effect of chemotherapy and radiation therapy. Not all chemotherapy drugs cause hair loss. The type of chemotherapy regimen and doses prescribed affect your chances of hair loss. Radiation therapy only causes hair loss in the area being treated. Hair loss typically starts 2 to 4 weeks after your treatments have started. You may experience thinning of the hair or complete hair loss. Hair loss caused by chemotherapy and radiation therapy is usually temporary. Regrowth of hair may start 6 to 8 weeks after completion of radiation therapy or after several cycles of chemotherapy. Your physician will inform you of your chances for hair loss before your treatments begin. The best way to deal with hair loss is to prepare for it before it happens. Here are some simple recommendations:

- Get a short, stylish haircut before beginning your treatments. This will prepare you for the change in your appearance due to hair loss.
- If you are considering a wig, see a wig stylist before your treatments begin. This will allow the stylist to match a wig to your natural color and texture.
- Ask your doctor for a prescription for a wig because some insurance companies pay for them.
- Once treatments begin use mild shampoo, pat the hair dry, and comb the hair carefully without tugging.
- Only use a hair dryer if necessary on low heat.
- Avoid hair dyes, rollers, curling irons, or permanents.
- Sleep on a satin pillow case to avoid friction between hair and scalp.

- Some patients feel more in control if they shave their heads completely so they do not have to deal with the hair falling out. (Remember, bald heads are in style!)
- Patients may choose to have their hair cut and made into a wig.
- Consider scarves, hats, and turbans in addition to, or instead of a wig.

# Preventing Lymphedema

Lymphatic fluid is a clear, colorless fluid that passes through the capillary walls into the tissues of your body. Lymph channels carry the lymphatic fluid first to lymph nodes, which filter out bacteria and other debris, and then back to the circulating blood. Lymph fluid is moved through the channels in the arms and legs by contraction of the muscles and valves, which prevent it from flowing backward. When surgery is performed on the lymph nodes in the armpit such as for breast cancer, the lymph flow may be slowed. Surgery on the lymph glands in the abdomen may slow the drainage of fluid from the legs. This might result in swelling of the arms or legs (lymphedema) depending on the area treated.

If you are a patient who has had combined surgery and radiation therapy to the lymph node region, you may be at an increased risk of developing lymphedema. You should notify your physician immediately if you develop swelling in the arm or leg. You may have an infection that requires prompt treatment. The most important way to combat lymphedema is to prevent its occurrence. Here are some simple recommendations:

* Keep the affected extremity clean with moisturizing soaps such as Dove.
* Keep the skin moisturized with lotions.
* Use an electric razor instead of a blade on the affected extremity or armpit if you are shaving this region.
* Protect the skin from the sun with sunscreen, at least SPF-15.
* Use insect repellents to prevent insect bites.
* Keep the extremity in an elevated position when you are resting; this lets gravity work to move the lymph fluid.

- Consider wearing a compression stocking on the extremity when flying in an airplane.
- Avoid hot showers, saunas, or steam rooms.
- Avoid excess alcohol and smoking.
- Do not have any blood pressure measurements, injections, blood draws, or vaccinations on the affected extremity.
- Maintain your ideal body weight.

## FOR THE ARM

- Wear rubber gloves when washing dishes.
- Wear protective gloves when doing work outside.
- Avoid carrying heavy objects with the affected arm.
- Carry heavy shoulder bags on the unaffected side.
- Do not get a manicure on the affected side.
- Do not wear a watch or jewelry on the affected side.

## FOR THE LEG

- Wear shoes or slippers around the house. Do not go barefoot.
- Consider having a podiatrist cut your toenails.
- Buy good, comfortable shoes.
- Wear work boots when doing chores outside.

*CancerTip*          **Managing Lymphedema**

Lymphedema is an accumulation of lymphatic fluid in the extremities due to alteration of normal lymphatic flow. The lymphatic drainage can be altered through surgery, radiation therapy, or direct blockage of the drainage by a tumor. Taking precautions to prevent lymphedema is the best initial approach in management. If lymphedema occurs, you should notify your physician immediately because you may need prompt antibiotic therapy. The treatment of chronic lymphedema requires a commitment to certain lifestyle modifications. You should see a physiatrist or physical therapist who specializes in the management of chronic lymphedema for appropriate therapeutic recommendations. There are therapies for the management of chronic lymphedema. These include:

- Keep the affected extremity higher than your heart to let gravity drain the accumulated fluid.
- Flexibility and strengthening exercises may help drain fluid through muscular contractions "milking" the fluid back through the extremity. You should discuss these exercises with your physical therapist or physician.
- Customized compression sleeves or elastic bandages applied in the proper manner may help prevent accumulation of fluid.
- Maintain your ideal body weight. Many overweight patients find that the lymphedema improves with weight loss.
- Reduce your salt and sugar intake to prevent fluid retention.
- Manual lymphatic drainage performed by a professional therapist with specialized training and certification.

- Pneumatic compression stockings may be prescribed for some patients.
- It is important to follow the recommendations to prevent lymphedema noted on the previous pages because these will help reduce the symptoms.

*CancerTip*          **Pain Management**

The goal of pain management for the cancer patient is the prevention or complete control of pain. There are many options available for the treatment of cancer-related pain. Most patients are treated with medications initially. Other treatments for pain may include surgery, radiation therapy, or nerve injections. Almost all patients have complete relief of pain with the appropriate management.

Cancer pain is usually caused by a tumor pressing against bones, nerves, or bodily organs. Cancer treatments can also cause pain and discomfort. Patients may have pain caused by things that have nothing to do with cancer such as muscle strains and arthritis.

The first step in the management of cancer pain is choosing the correct pain medication. There may be a period of trial and error while your physician attempts to find the right medication and dosage for you. There are large varieties of medications that range in strength from over-the-counter medications such as aspirin to strong prescription medications such as morphine. Medications may be short acting and taken on an "as-needed" basis, or long acting to suppress any pain before it occurs. Pain medications may be given as pills, liquids, suppositories, skin patches, or injections.

There are some nondrug treatments of pain that are effective for some patients. Guided imagery can be a very effective and soothing technique. Breathing and relaxation exercises can also help many patients. Transcutaneous electrical nerve stimulation (TENS) units may be prescribed in specific circumstances. Hot or cold packs may also provide symptomatic relief of discomfort.

There are some important points to remember when dealing with cancer pain that include:

- Take charge and become an active participant in the health-care team.
- Be honest with your physicians and nurses about your pain.
- Keep a diary of the times you are in pain.
- Score your pain on a scale of 0 to 10 (0= no pain, 10= excruciating pain).
- Note how much medication you are taking and the time you take your pills.
- Always let your physician know if the pain is worsening or you develop bowel or bladder problems.
- Make sure you are on appropriate medications to prevent constipation if you are taking any narcotics for pain control.
- Take your medications as prescribed. Do not wait until the pain is unbearable. It is easier to prevent pain or relieve it when it starts than to wait until it gets bad.
- Do not worry that you will become "hooked" or "addicted" to your pain medication. Studies have shown this outcome is very rare with cancer patients.
- Contact your nurse or doctor if your pain medication is not working.

# Skin Care and Radiation Therapy

One of the most common side effects of radiation therapy is skin irritation in the area of the body that is being treated. The skin reaction can range from very mild redness and dryness (similar to a sunburn) to severe desquamation (peeling) of the skin in some rare patients. With modern radiation techniques, many patients can be spared significant symptoms related to the skin. There are, however, some instances where full treatment to the skin is required.

Always let your nurse or doctor know if your skin is becoming irritated. Most patients start with some redness and dryness to the skin 2 to 3 weeks into treatment. This can progress to peeling and ultimately moist desquamation with oozing of fluid in the area. There are effective topical medications available for radiation-induced skin irritation. Typically, the nurses in the radiation oncology department are the most experienced in dealing with skin reactions. There are some rare instances in which radiation therapy must be placed on hold to allow for some skin healing, but this is a decision that must be made by the treating oncologist.

Skin reactions can be magnified in those patients who are receiving chemotherapy along with radiation therapy. There is also a reaction known as the "radiation recall phenomenon" that can occur with specific chemotherapy agents, particularly Adriamycin. In this phenomenon, skin may completely heal after the radiation treatments only to have the same skin reaction occur some time later with the start of Adriamycin therapy.

There are some precautions that patients can take to minimize skin irritation during radiation treatments:

- Wash only the skin in the treatment area with mild soaps such as Dove.
- Use a mild shampoo, such as baby shampoo, if the head is being treated.
- When using a towel, pat the area dry instead of rubbing.
- If you must shave in the treated area, use an electric razor to prevent cuts.
- Avoid using shaving lotions or scented creams.
- Do not use perfumes, deodorants, or makeup in the treated area.
- Always check with your nurse or doctor before using creams or lotions on the skin. Samples of safe topical medications are usually available in the radiation clinic.
- Avoid using heating pads and ice packs on the skin in the treated area.
- Use only paper tape with dressings applied to the treated area.
- Wear loose-fitting clothing that does not rub on the skin in the radiated area.
- Avoid sun exposure in the treated area (e.g., use hats, thick clothing, and umbrellas).

*CancerTip* **Weight Loss**

One of the most common symptoms of cancer and a frequent side effect of cancer treatment is unintentional weight loss. Many patients experience a loss of appetite and significant reduction in their weight. Cancer can cause a wasting syndrome called cachexia. This clinical syndrome includes weight loss, decreased appetite, fatigue, and significant alterations in activities of daily living. It is multifactorial in nature and associated with mechanical factors, changes in taste, chemical factors, and psychological factors.

Many of the treatments for cancer, including chemotherapy and radiation therapy, may decrease a patient's appetite. Patients need to maintain their nutrition to allow normal tissue repair after aggressive cancer treatments. There can be significant problems with healing if the patient has poor nutrition. Poor nutrition can alter the ability of a patient to tolerate a specific treatment and cause adjustment in the dose of chemotherapy and radiation treatments. This could ultimately decrease the effectiveness of a particular therapy.

Although many patients may lose their appetite, they should keep a regular meal schedule. Small, frequent meals are much more tolerable than three large meals each day. Patients should not try to force themselves to eat their favorite foods. They may just develop an aversion to them when they are feeling better. Avoid spicy, hot, and fried foods. Try to eat foods that are soft, easily swallowed, and are high in calories such as milkshakes, eggs, creamy soups, pastas, and mashed potatoes. Nausea can be controlled effectively with appropriate medications and prevention strategies.

There are many commercial liquid supplements on the market today including Ensure, Boost, Carnation, and Sustacal. These supplements can be used to help increase caloric intake. Just to maintain the weight of an average person, six to seven cans are required if no other food is consumed. Patients who are receiving radiation therapy to the head and neck region or esophagus sometimes need temporary feeding tubes placed in the stomach or intestine to maintain nutrition during treatment.

Sometimes a medication called Megace will help stimulate the appetite in cancer patients. Megace is supplied in a liquid suspension (40 mg/mL), and the recommended dose is 800 mg/day. It usually takes 1 to 2 weeks before a patient experiences an increase in their appetite. It can take a few weeks before there is significant weight gain. The most common side effects include fluid retention and loss of libido in men. There is also an increased risk of developing blood clots. The medication is relatively expensive, so patients should make sure it is covered under their prescription plan. If a patient does not have prescription medication coverage, they may qualify for special assistance programs.

Patients should discuss strategies to maintain their weight and adequate nutritional status with their oncologist. Also, meeting with a nutritionist who is experienced with cancer patients can be very beneficial.

# SECTION III   SEXUALITY ISSUES

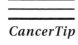

*CancerTip*

# Dealing With Vaginal Discomfort During Intercourse After Cancer Treatment

Vaginal discomfort during intercourse is a common complaint of women after treatment for cancer. Radiation therapy to the pelvis, chemotherapy-induced menopause, or restrictions on the use of estrogen replacement in postmenopausal women may all affect the ability to enjoy sexual relations. This discomfort may be caused by vaginal dryness or a loss of stretch of the vaginal tissues. Patients who receive radiation therapy to the pelvic region or radiation implants may need to use vaginal dilators on a regular basis to prevent scar tissue and closure of the vagina. Patients who are postmenopausal may experience a decrease in natural lubrication of the vagina. There are some effective treatments available. These treatments include:

- Using extra lubrication to reduce pain.
- Use only water-based lubricants.
- Many women prefer lubricants such as Astroglide, Moist Again, the Women's Health Institutes Lubricating Gel, and Probe to other products because they spread easily and last longer.
- Avoid petroleum-based lubricants, particularly if your partner is using condoms that can be damaged with this type of lubrication.
- Avoid scented lubricants because these agents may irritate the genital tissues.
- Use lubricants during foreplay and spread generously over the labia, the clitoris, and into the vagina. Also, spread lubrication on any object that will enter the vagina.
- Keep lubricants close to the bed or anywhere sexual activity may occur.

- Consider using Replens, which is designed to moisturize the walls of the vagina. It is used about three times per week at bedtime.
- If your radiation oncologist has prescribed vaginal dilators, make sure you use them as instructed.

*CancerTip*

# Treatments for Erectile Dysfunction After Cancer Treatment

Many men may have difficulty obtaining or maintaining erections after various forms of cancer treatment. Surgery and radiation therapy to the pelvic area, hormonal therapy, chemotherapy, and various medications may all significantly impact a man's ability to obtain or maintain an erection. Erectile dysfunction can cause significant anxiety for the man and his partner.

Because this is a common complaint after cancer treatment, you should feel at ease that your physician has seen many patients with similar problems. You should not hesitate to discuss these concerns with your physician. After a thorough history and physical examination, your doctor may recommend specific testing or changes in your medications. There are medical treatments to help patients restore and maintain erections. Only your physician can determine if you will benefit from a specific treatment. These treatments may include the following:

- Vacuum Constrictive Devices (VCDs)—This is a pump that you place over the penis. As air is pumped out of the cylinder, blood is drawn into the penis to produce an erection. A ring slides over the base of the penis to keep the blood in the tissues to maintain an erection for up to half an hour.
- Penile Injections—Drugs that promote blood flow may be injected into the side of the penis. The most common drug used for injection is prostaglandin $E_1$ (Caverject). The medication typically needs to be adjusted to the correct dose based on the time the erection is maintained.

- Muse System—This system also uses prostaglandin $E_1$. Instead of an injection, a small suppository is placed into the urethra using a specialized applicator.
- Penile Prosthesis (Implants)—There are various types of penile prostheses that a man can consider. Some are malleable rods that are placed in the penis. Most men now use different types of inflatable prostheses.
- Sex Therapy—This is recommended for patients with anxiety-based erection problems. Typically, the patient and his partner are both involved in the therapy sessions.
- Drug Therapy—See the next section.
- There are advantages and disadvantages with each type of treatment. There are also different side effects for each treatment. If you are experiencing erectile dysfunction you should discuss the pros and cons of each treatment option with your physician.

# Viagra—A New Treatment for Erectile Dysfunction

The Food and Drug Administration recently approved sildenafil citrate (Viagra), the first oral pill to treat impotence. Viagra affects the response to sexual stimulation by enhancing the smooth muscle relaxant effects of a chemical called nitric oxide. This allows increased blood flow into certain areas of the penis leading to an erection.

Viagra was evaluated in numerous trials involving 3,700 men with various degrees of impotence associated with spinal cord injury, history of prostate surgery, diabetes, and no identifiable cause of organic impotence. In all preapproval trials, men who took Viagra reported success more often than did men on placebo, and the rates of success increased with the dose. Across all trials, Viagra improved the erections of 43% of prostate cancer patients treated with radical prostatectomy patients compared with 15% receiving a placebo.

Viagra is available only by prescription from your physician. The recommended dose is 50 mg taken 1 hour before sexual activity. The dose may be adjusted by a physician depending on the patient's response. The drug should not be taken more than once a day. Viagra has no effect in the absence of sexual stimulation.

There are some precautions and contraindications to the use of Viagra. Men who have conditions that may cause sustained erections (priapism) such as sickle cell anemia, leukemia, or multiple myeloma should not take Viagra. The drug should not be used in combination with organic nitrates such as nitroglycerin patches or tabs placed under the tongue because the combination may lower blood pressure. Also, those patients who have Peyronie's disease may need to take

Viagra with caution. As with any medication, Viagra can inter-act with other prescription and over-the-counter medications. Anyone considering Viagra should discuss all of their medica-tions with their physician. Viagra has not been studied in com-bination with other treatments for erectile dysfunction, so its use in combination with these other methods is not recom-mended outside of a clinical research study.

Viagra seems to be well tolerated, with the most common side effects being headache, flushing, and indigestion. Some patients report changes in vision, principally color perception. As with any new medication, more side effects may be reported with the increased use of the medication.

After various forms of cancer treatment, many men have difficulty getting or maintaining erections. Surgery and radia-tion therapy to the pelvic area, hormonal therapy, chemother-apy, and medications may all significantly impact a man's abil-ity to obtain erections. Erectile dysfunction can cause significant anxiety for the man and his partner. There are many treatments available for erectile dysfunction in the cancer pa-tient. Viagra may be a viable treatment for some patients, but this needs to be determined on an individual basis.

# SECTION IV

# PHYSICIAN AND PATIENT INTERACTION

# Finding an Oncologist

A diagnosis of cancer can immediately turn a person's life up-side down. Things begin to spiral out of control, and one feels as if he or she has lost command of both body and life. Autopilot goes on. It is exactly at this time that one of the most important decisions needs to be made—"Who will be my oncologist?"

One of the first surprises that many cancer patients find is that they are really choosing a whole team of people, not just one oncologist. There may be a surgeon, medical oncologist, and radiation oncologist all intimately involved in an individual's cancer care. There are also a slew of nurses, nurse practitioners, technicians, and other support staff that are important members of the team. This may make the task of choosing the right team seem daunting. However, especially at institutions that treat cancer on a regular basis, many cancer teams are already assembled. Physicians who work well together usually treat the same patients and refer patients to each other. Also, these physicians tend to put together a team with a "personality" similar to their own. You need to think of your physician as the quarterback; the leader of the team, but not more important than any of the other positions on the field. Quarterbacks try to surround themselves with good players, so everything runs smoothly and correctly. The quarterback also needs to choose players that he can trust to do the job correctly so the entire team works efficiently. Fortunately, this decision process may not be as difficult as it seems if you follow some basic guidelines.

- You are in control. The final decisions are yours. You are the most important part of your healthcare team.

- Choose your quarterback, the rest will usually fall into place. Ask your primary care physician for a recommendation— your primary care physician has sent numerous patients to oncologists. They will typically know the oncologist on a professional level. They will have also had reports from the patients they have sent in the past on the quality of care that they received.
- Comprehensive Cancer Centers typically have a team approach to the treatment of malignancies. You may consider a consultation at such a facility, and ask to meet an entire team of physicians there.
- You may want to speak with people that have a similar diagnosis and have already gone through treatment, and then ask them for a recommendation.
- Contact your local American Cancer Society (ACS)—Your local ACS should have a list of the regional cancer centers and facilities that deal with your diagnosis.
- Nurses—Nurses can be a great resource. Most have contacts with other nurses who may work with oncologists. They can typically give you the "inside scoop" on what a physician is really like.
- Support groups—Sometimes local support groups can be helpful. You may find people who have already experienced a similar cancer diagnosis.
- Internet—The Internet can be a great resource to obtain information and locate facilities in your area. Just remember, many excellent private practice oncologists do not have their own website, so this resource should be used in conjunction with the previous recommendations.

# Becoming Involved in Clinical Research Trials

There are clinical research trials that are ongoing for almost every type of cancer. Clinical trials are experiments to determine the value of specific treatments. There are international, national, and institutional research trials. Each clinical research trial must be approved by an Institutional Review Board (IRB), which is composed of physicians, researchers, and even people not involved in medicine. The IRB decides if the study is reasonable, appropriately designed, and safe for the patient population. Anyone considering joining a clinical research trial must be fully informed about the trial details, benefits, and risks. All patients must sign informed consent. Trials may involve chemotherapy, radiation therapy, surgery, new experimental modalities, or any combination of these treatments.

There are different types of clinical trials that are divided into the following phases:

Phase I clinical trials attempt to determine the dose of a drug that is appropriate. Phase I trials typically include patients who have advanced disease, which is resistant to standard treatments. The dose is typically increased as additional patients are added on the study to determine the maximum tolerated dose.

Phase II trials attempt to measure the biologic response of a particular tumor to a specific treatment. Typically, patients with a tumor for which there is not an effective therapy are included in phase II trials of single agents. Combination regimens may also be evaluated in phase II trials. The goal of a combination regimen phase II trial is to ensure that the treatment is feasible, safe, and promising enough before expanding to the next phase.

Phase III trials are designed to compare an experimental treatment to an accepted standard treatment and evaluate endpoints such as survival and symptom control. These trials typically are performed in multiinstitutional settings that include physicians from the community.

Clinical research trials are extremely important in expanding treatment options in all cancers. The treatments that are available today are a result of the participation of other cancer patients in clinical research trials. We are constantly trying to identify better treatments to cure cancer. There are also studies to identify less toxic treatments or agents, which can protect the normal tissues and minimize side effects of treatment. Clinical research trials are very rewarding for both the patient and the physician. The patient may benefit from new treatment options and help future cancer patients in their fight against this disease. OncoLink strongly recommends that patients discuss any clinical research trials for which they may be eligible with their oncologist.

# Preparing for Your First Oncology Consultation

If you are diagnosed with cancer, you will be referred to an oncologist for evaluation and treatment recommendations. There are actually a number of different types of oncologists. You may see a surgical oncologist who specializes in the surgical resection of cancers. You may also be referred to a radiation oncologist who specializes in the treatment of cancer using radiation therapy. The third type of oncologist is a medical oncologist. These physicians specialize in the use of chemotherapy in the treatment of cancer. All of these physicians work closely together, and there are overlapping roles in the treatment of most cancers.

Going to your first oncology consultation can create significant anxiety. There are many questions to be asked by both the patient and physician. A number of things can be done by the patient to prepare for the oncology consultation that can make the whole experience easier. It is important that the patient become an active member of the healthcare team. Here are some simple recommendations:

- Forward all of your recent medical records including operative reports, pathology reports, and radiology reports to your oncologist.
- Make sure you have any necessary referrals before seeing your oncologist.
- Bring all of your recent radiology films including x-ray studies, mammograms, computed tomography (CT) scans, magnetic resonance imaging (MRI) scans, and ultrasound studies to your oncology appointment if these examinations were performed at another location.

- Bring a family member or close friend to the appointment to take notes and help ask questions.
- Consider bringing a tape recorder and asking permission to tape the conversation with your physician so you can review the details of your conversation.
- Write down questions before your consultation.
- Bring pathology slides for review if a surgery diagnosing cancer was done at another institution.
- Consider having your consultation at a multidisciplinary clinic if this is available in your area.
- Make sure your oncologist's secretary has received all of the necessary information before your visit.
- If you are bringing radiology films to your consultation from an outside location, you may wish to arrive early or drop these films off for review before your appointment.
- Bring a list of all of your medications and allergies to medications.
- Bring a list of the physicians and the addresses where you want reports of the consultation sent.
- Make sure you bring your health insurance identification card if you have one.
- Get all of your questions answered before leaving.
- Get an appointment for follow-up.
- Make sure your have the phone number of your oncologist's secretary.
- Try not to become frustrated if additional blood tests, x-ray studies, or other procedures are necessary before getting a final recommendation.
- Keep a journal of tests, procedures, and treatments that includes the date, location, and physician involved.

# Keep Your Follow-up Appointments

Your cancer care continues even after you have completed your planned course of treatment. Any physician who participated actively in your care should continue to see you for routine check-ups. This may include your medical oncologist, radiation oncologist, and surgeon. Follow-up appointments will be frequent initially. As time passes, the intervals between visits will be lengthened at the discretion of your physicians. You should contact your physicians immediately if there is any change in your medical condition. If you move a great distance from the location in which you initially received treatment, it is important you find qualified physicians in your local area to continue your follow-up care. There are some very important reasons to keep your follow-up appointments. These include:

- Management of any side effects from your cancer treatments.
- Your physicians must follow you closely for the development of any late complications of treatment.
- Early detection of any cancer recurrence that may be amenable to treatment.
- Because any cancer patient is at increased risk of a second malignancy, it is imperative that you are closely followed so that (if they occur) these cancers are identified at an early stage.
- Regular cancer screening at appropriate intervals.
- Detection of premalignant changes and the institution of treatment before cancer develops.
- Management of medications that may decrease the risk of cancer recurrence and a second malignancy (e.g., tamoxifen in breast cancer patients).
- Discussion of any new concerns that may arise.

# ONCOLOGIC EMERGENCIES

*CancerTip*  **Neutropenic Fever**

Neutropenic fever is an oncologic emergency. If you are receiving chemotherapy, you are at particular risk of developing neutropenic fevers. Neutropenia occurs when the number of your white blood cells, specifically the neutrophil population, becomes dangerously low. Neutrophils are important in fighting bacterial infections and act as one of the body's important defense mechanisms. Without adequate numbers of neutrophils, the body can be quickly overwhelmed by a bacterial infection. This is one of the reasons that your blood counts are followed so closely when you are receiving chemotherapy.

The first sign of an infection may be a fever. It is important that you keep a functioning thermometer available. Do not take your temperature rectally, because this may introduce bacteria into your blood stream. An oral thermometer or the newer thermometer that measures your temperature from your ear canal is adequate. If you have a temperature greater than 100.5°F, you should notify your physician immediately.

If you are unable to contact your physician within a few minutes by telephone, proceed to the nearest emergency room. If you have been informed that your white blood count is low and a fever develops, you must go to an emergency room immediately. Neutropenic fever may cause serious effects, including death, very quickly.

Prompt initiation of broad-spectrum intravenous antibiotics is mandatory in the case of neutropenic fever. Do not delay in getting to a hospital. A fever with a low neutrophil count is a true emergency!

**Spinal Cord Compression**

Spinal cord compression is considered an oncologic emergency that requires prompt intervention. The spinal cord runs within the vertebral column and extends from the brain stem to the lumbar vertebral body level (low back). Tumors that are growing within the spine can place pressure on the spinal cord. Because the cord is circled by bone, a tumor growing within the spinal canal causes compression of the spinal cord against bone. The nerves can be irritated and damaged if prompt treatment is not obtained.

A variety of tumors may cause spinal cord compression. Primary spinal tumors are relatively rare in the adult with an incidence of 1,800 to 2,000 per year in the United States. Metastatic tumors to the spine have an incidence of approximately 22,000 per year. The most common tumors to spread and cause spinal cord compression are lung, breast, and prostate cancer.

Any time a cancer patient develops new back pain, spinal cord compression is a concern. The symptoms of spinal cord compression correspond directly to the area of the spinal cord that is being compressed. Back pain is the most common presenting symptom. However, patients may also complain of weakness in the extremities and sensory changes. These symptoms can progress to loss of bowel and bladder control, loss of sensation below the level of the tumor, and paralysis. Progression of symptoms can be relatively rapid, thus prompt evaluation and treatment is mandatory.

How is spinal cord compression diagnosed? A physician performs a complete history and physical examination, with special attention to the neurologic examination. If the physician is suspicious that spinal cord compression may be present, an emergent magnetic resonance imaging (MRI) scan of the spine is performed. If the MRI confirms spinal cord compression, prompt treatment is initiated.

Treatment may include surgery, radiation therapy, and steroids. A neurosurgeon may recommend removal (decompression) of the mass pushing on the spinal cord. However, there are multiple factors that affect the decision to perform surgery, which are beyond the scope of this book. If surgery is an option, radiation therapy may be given 1 to 3 weeks after surgery to prevent local recurrence of the tumor. If surgical decompression is not an option, external beam radiation therapy may be used to treat the tumor. Steroids may be used to decrease the swelling and pressure on the spinal cord. Chemotherapy may be used in some rare instances as primary management of spinal cord compression.

Any cancer patient who develops new back pain and/or neurologic symptoms should notify their physician immediately. Prompt evaluation and treatment may prevent catastrophic results such as loss of bowel and bladder function and paralysis.

## *CancerTip*    Superior Vena Cava Syndrome

Superior vena cava (SVC) syndrome is considered a situation that requires emergency evaluation and treatment. The syndrome is caused by compression of the major vein that drains the blood from the head, neck, upper chest, and arms. This may cause shortness of breath, facial and neck swelling, arm swelling, and cough. It can progress very rapidly to obstruction of the airway and cause a patient to be placed on a respirator to assist with breathing.

Cancer is the most common cause of SVC syndrome. Lung cancer, lymphoma, and germ cell tumors of the chest are most commonly associated with SVC syndrome. Any cancer that has spread to the lymph nodes in the chest may cause compression of the superior vena cava. Some patients present with SVC syndrome as their first symptom of cancer. It can also be caused by some noncancerous conditions including goiter, aortic aneurysm, and inflammation of the mediastinum. Rarely, central venous catheters can cause clot to form and contribute to a SVC syndrome.

How is SVC syndrome diagnosed? Your physician will perform a complete history and physical examination. They will look specifically for signs associated with SVC syndrome. A chest x-ray study and computed tomography (CT) scan of the chest may be recommended. The CT scan can show compression of the SVC very clearly.

SVC syndrome caused by cancer requires prompt initiation of treatment. This condition can progress rapidly. Patients already with a diagnosis of cancer may be placed on steroids to help relieve the swelling. Radiation therapy directed at the mass causing the obstruction might give relief rapidly.

Chemotherapy may be used for the treatment of SVC when the tumor is considered responsive to specific medications. Rarely, surgery may be considered as primary management of SVC syndrome.

For those patients without a cancer diagnosis who present with a mass in the chest and clinical SVC syndrome, a biopsy must be obtained to confirm a malignancy. If treatment with steroids or radiation is initiated before a biopsy, it can be very difficult to obtain an accurate diagnosis. This could dramatically influence subsequent cancer management.

SVC syndrome is a true cancer emergency. Any new swelling in the face and arms associated with shortness of breath should be reported to your oncologist immediately.

# ALTERNATIVE MEDICINE

*CancerTip*

# Conventional Versus Unconventional Cancer Treatments

What is alternative medicine? How about complementary treatments? Is this conventional medicine? How about unconventional treatments? These terms are often used without explaining the definitions. With the increased popularity of unconventional medical treatments, these terms are being used more and more. Here is a guide to help with the confusing jargon.

Conventional cancer therapies consist of those forms of cancer treatment that are widely practiced and have been proven beneficial in clinical research trials. These may include surgery, chemotherapy, radiation therapy, or hormonal therapy. These treatments are used in mainstream cancer centers throughout the world.

Unconventional cancer therapies are basically any approaches to the diagnosis, treatment, and care of the cancer patient that fall outside conventional cancer treatments. Many different categories of unconventional therapies have been described, including psychological techniques, specialized diets, herbal therapies, spiritual healers, traditional cultural techniques, and pharmacologic treatments. Unconventional treatments have not been proved to cure cancer in scientific research trials. Some treatments have been shown to be beneficial in helping patients with the side effects of their conventional medical treatments. Unconventional medical therapies fall under two broad categories: complementary versus alternative.

Complementary cancer treatments are those unconventional cancer therapies used in conjunction with conventional medical treatments (such as acupuncture and guided imagery used for nausea caused by chemotherapy).

Alternative cancer treatments are those unconventional cancer therapies that are used instead of conventional medical therapies.

Always discuss any unconventional medical treatments that you are considering with your physician. Although these therapies can be helpful, many can interact with your body and make it difficult for you to complete your conventional medical treatments that have been proved to cure cancer.

*CancerTip*

# Watch Out for a Hoax

Unconventional medical treatments for cancer are gaining increasing exposure to the public through television, the Internet, and magazines. Some unconventional therapies may one day prove to help cancer patients. These therapies are classified as "alternative" or "unconventional" because they have not been proved to benefit cancer patients in controlled clinical trials. It is a challenge to differentiate those techniques that offer promise from those that are hoaxes.

Many individuals claim that natural products are better to combat cancer than conventional treatments such as chemotherapy, radiation therapy, and surgery. Poison ivy is natural, but most patients would not go and rub it intentionally all over their body. Rattlesnakes are natural, but most patients would not try to be bitten by one. Obviously, just because something is natural does not mean it is effective and safe. It is true that many of the therapies used today were discovered in nature. These have been isolated, standardized, and purified. They have also been rigorously tested in controlled clinical trials to establish the effectiveness of the agent and its side effect profile.

Cancer patients are prime targets for unscrupulous individuals who attempt to gain financially from the misfortunes of others. Always remember that if a treatment sounds too good to be true, it may be a hoax. Here are some classic signs of a hoax that should place the cancer patient on the alert:

- The treatment is a "secret" that only specific individuals can provide.
- Patients are told not to use conventional medical treatment.

- The treatment promises a cure for almost all cancers or medical conditions.
- The treatment is only promoted in the mass media such as the Internet, talk shows, and books instead of reputable scientific journals.
- The promoters claim that they are persecuted by the medical establishment.
- Advertisements for the treatment claim to "cleanse the body of poisons and toxins."
- The treatment will help the patient by "strengthening the immune system."
- Testimonials and case reports are used to promote a specific treatment or product.
- Catch phrases such as "nontoxic," "no side effects," and "painless" are used.
- The promoters attack the medical community.

If you are considering an alternative or complementary treatment, be cautious and aware of any of the above-mentioned claims. Always tell your doctor if you are considering any such treatment. Certain treatments may be helpful, but others may interfere with your traditional treatments.

*Cancer Tip*    **Acupuncture**

Acupuncture has been practiced in China for more than 5,000 years. Acupuncture may be recommended for various conditions, but pain or nausea and vomiting are of greatest interest for cancer patients. The Japanese have also used shiatsu, or acupressure, which is pressure applied to designated points in the body.

Acupuncturists use needles that are hair thin and vary in length from less than 1 inch to several inches. The needles are usually made of stainless steel or copper. They are placed about 1/4-inch deep and are gently twisted by hand. The needles may be stimulated with a weak electrical current or heat. Many patients describe a tingling sensation and feel a sense of heaviness in the area the needles are placed. Some say it feels like a mosquito bite.

Much of the evidence in support of acupuncture is anecdotal. It has been reported as effective for pain, alcoholism, drug abuse, smoking, gastrointestinal disorders, hot flashes, and asthma, just to name a few conditions. There have been studies suggesting patients undergoing chemotherapy experience relief of nausea after acupuncture. There is also some evidence suggesting patients with pain related to cancer need fewer pain medications after acupuncture.

So how does acupuncture work? The classic acupuncture teaching states that a life force called qi dominates every organism and flows along interconnected meridians through the body and crosses at specific points. The meridians surface at various locations denoting the acupuncture points. The opposing forces of yin and yang must be in balance before qi can get the body's vital functions to work normally. The imbalance causes an accumulation of lactic acid in the muscles. Stimulating the acupoints is said to dissipate the lactic acid and restore the yin-yang balance and the flow of qi.

Scientists in the western world have found no evidence to support the existence of qi, yin, yang, or meridians. They have found that stimulation of acupoints with needles causes the release of natural opiates called endorphins. These substances are released within the nervous system and reduce the perception of pain. It has also been shown that the acupoints have a greater concentration of nerve endings than do other locations on the body.

Acupuncture may benefit some patients on an individual basis. It is difficult to make broad recommendations on its applicability due to the lack of clinical trials evaluating this alternative medical technique. There are studies in progress that will hopefully shed additional light on the benefits of acupuncture. Here are a few words of caution to the cancer patient who is considering acupuncture:

- Only visit an acupuncturist who is properly licensed. In the United States, a license is required in all 50 states.
- Do not let an acupuncturist place needles in a cancerous mass or lump because this may promote spread of the tumor.
- Do not have acupuncture performed if you are neutropenic (have a low white blood cell count) because you are at a very high risk of infections that can be introduced with the needles.
- Do not have acupuncture performed if you are thrombocytopenic (have a low platelet count) because you are at an increased risk of bleeding.

- Make sure that the needles are new and disposable so you are not exposed to human immunodeficiency virus (HIV), hepatitis, or other infections.
- Always let your physician know that you are considering acupuncture before you start receiving the treatments. There may be specific cautions associated with your medical condition.

*CancerTip*  **Green Tea**

Green tea has been promoted as an agent to prevent the development of cancer. It purported to contain antioxidants that reduce the risk of some cancers, particularly those of the gastrointestinal tract. Claims have also been made that it can lower cholesterol and triglyceride levels and lower the risk of cardiovascular disease.

It originates from the same plant as black tea, but the leaves are prepared differently. Unlike black tea, the leaves are steamed to prevent oxidation of the active agents. Green tea is very popular in China, Japan, and India. People generally drink three cups per day to promote health. The taste of green tea is very different from black tea, which has limited its popularity in the western world. It is available in grocery stores and sold in tea bags or as dried herb.

There are a number of retrospective studies performed in Japan and China that indicate individuals who drink green tea have a lower incidence of cancer. There are also claims that those who develop cancer tend to do so at an older age. Green tea has been shown to inhibit tumor growth in test tubes in some studies. However, there are no prospective randomized studies proving its efficacy in humans.

Because green tea originates from the same plant as black tea, caffeine is contained within the tea. Side effects are related to the caffeine and consist of insomnia, palpitations, nervousness, and headaches. Those patients who suffer from migraine headaches, irregular heartbeats, and anxiety disorders should avoid large amounts of any beverage with caffeine. Pregnant or nursing women should also avoid large amounts of caffeine.

If you are considering using an alternative or complementary treatment such as green tea, always discuss it with your doctor. There are numerous studies evaluating the use of green tea for the prevention of cancer. Until these studies are completed, final recommendation regarding the use of green tea cannot be made.

*CancerTip*

# Herbal Remedies May Affect the Screening Test for Prostate Cancer

It is estimated that 198,100 men will be diagnosed with prostate cancer in the year 2001. Most patients are screened for prostate cancer with a blood test that detects a substance called prostate specific antigen (PSA). Screening for PSA has been so successful that most cases of prostate cancer are picked up by this screening test and patients are being diagnosed at earlier stages of disease.

With the increased use of herbal therapies, it has been found that a number of these natural supplements may affect the PSA blood test. Most of these herbs are touted as "supporters of prostate health." You can see the advertisements on television, read them in the press, and hear them on the radio. Because these herbal therapies are natural supplements, they are not regulated by the Food and Drug Administration (FDA). The only requirement is that they do not claim effectiveness against a particular disease. So the manufacturers use vague claims such as "supporting male wellness" or "supporting prostate health." Herbal therapies that may lower the PSA blood test include Saw Palmetto, PC-SPES, Lycopene, and other phytoestrogen combinations.

These natural therapies are medications. They can affect a number of processes within the body. Because they fall under the heading of supplements, they do not undergo the rigorous scientific testing expected of medications approved by the FDA. In addition, because they are not regulated, supplements from different companies may have completely different content. In fact, frequently there are variations of concentration of herbal batches from the same company.

Many men take these supplements without knowing some of these herbs can affect the PSA blood test used to detect prostate cancer early. There is a possibility some of these medications will cause a delay in diagnosis of prostate cancer. It is important for your physician to know if you are taking these therapies because they may place less reliance on the traditional values used for normal PSA. Also, they may place more importance on regular prostate physical examinations. If there is a slight trend upward in the PSA, even when it is in the normal range, your physician may be more likely to recommend a biopsy to rule out a cancer. The bottom line is that the normal thresholds used by physicians for further evaluation need to be changed when patients are using therapies that may cause a decrease in the PSA.

For those patients treated for prostate cancer with surgery or radiation, using herbal therapies without the knowledge of your physician may cause them to make false assumptions of effectiveness of a conventional therapy. This may cause a delay in the evaluation of recurrence of prostate cancer and the institution of appropriate therapy.

Always discuss the use of unconventional medical therapies with your physician. This will allow informed recommendations to be made for management of your condition. It is hoped that we will gain more insight into these therapies with rigorous scientific testing.

*CancerTip*        **Lycopene**

Lycopene is primarily derived from tomatoes and in the same family of compounds as beta-carotene. It is considered a strong antioxidant. A number of population-based studies have suggested increased tomato intake or elevated blood lycopene levels may reduce the incidence of prostate cancer, lung cancer, and stomach cancer. A recent review of the literature on lycopene revealed that 72 population-based studies have been performed. Fifty-seven of these studies reported a lower risk of cancer with increased intake of tomatoes or higher blood lycopene levels. Thirty-five of these studies were considered significant by statistical analysis.

A recent study evaluated the blood levels of the five major carotenoids in patients with prostate cancer and compared these levels with those of cancer-free subjects of the same age. Lycopene was the only major antioxidant found in significantly lower levels in the cancer patients than control subjects. Plasma lycopene levels were strongly related to lower prostate cancer risk. A preliminary study that was recently reported at a major scientific meeting suggested that lycopene may affect the growth of cancer cells.

This recent information has made lycopene a hot topic, particularly for the treatment of prostate cancer. It must be mentioned that none of these studies offer definitive proof that lycopene should be used as a treatment for prostate cancer. Population-based studies can imply only associations and do not support a cause-and-effect relationship. Thus, there is not enough information available to make definitive recommendations on the utilization of lycopene. Clinical research studies are ongoing to evaluate the effectiveness of lycopene in controlled clinical trials. However, there is no evidence that increasing the intake of tomatoes or tomato-based products has a detrimental effect on the health of patients.

Make sure to inform your physicians if you are taking or are considering taking lycopene. There is evidence that lycopene may affect the PSA blood test used in screening for prostate cancer. It is important physicians know when a patient is taking lycopene so that proper decisions are made based on the PSA test results.

*CancerTip*    # Megadose Vitamin C

Alternative and complementary medical techniques are gaining popularity in the treatment of cancer. One such treatment is the use of megadose vitamin C. Linus Pauling and Ewan Cameron wrote *Cancer and Vitamin C* in 1979. They claimed that high doses of vitamin C could significantly improve survival in cancer patients. It was recommended that cancer patients take 10,000 mg of vitamin C daily based on their research.

They reported a study of 100 terminal cancer patients treated with megadose vitamin C who had a significant survival advantage when compared with historical controls. Review of the study demonstrated significant bias and statistical problems. The "terminal"cancer patients who were treated with vitamin C all came from Cameron's practice, whereas the historical controls were "terminal" patients who came from other practices in the area. It is conceivable that significant selection bias occurred between Cameron's patients given vitamin C and the patients of other physicians who were not offered any additional treatments.

Because of Pauling's reputation, the Mayo Clinic performed a prospective randomized study to evaluate vitamin C. Patients with advanced cancer were randomized to 10 g of vitamin C versus a placebo. The study was criticized by Pauling for poor design, and the study was repeated twice. Each time the study was adjusted with consideration of the criticisms of Pauling. Similar results were obtained in all three studies performed at the Mayo Clinic. There was no difference in patient comfort or survival in any of the studies.

Side effects of megadose vitamin C include diarrhea, renal stones, iron overload, and abdominal cramping. The book *Vitamin C and Cancer* remains on the shelves of bookstores throughout the country. There are ardent supporters of megadose vitamin C despite the strong scientific evidence refuting its use in the treatment of cancer.

Based on the current scientific literature, megadose vitamin C is not recommended for the treatment of cancer.

*CancerTip*          **Macrobiotic Diet**

Various dietary regimens have been promoted for both the prevention and treatment of cancer. The macrobiotic diet was first described by George Ohsawa (1893 to 1966). He developed a diet consisting of 10 stages, with each stage more restrictive than the previous stage. The final stage consisted of only rice and water. The American Medical Association and various governmental health agencies opposed the macrobiotic diet owing to its restrictive nature. In fact, there were a number of reports of health problems and even deaths.

The diet has subsequently been modified and is regaining popularity in the United States. It generally consists of 50% to 60% whole grains, 20% to 25% vegetables, 5% to10% beans and sea vegetables, and 5% soups. Some variations of the diet allow small amounts of fish. There may be variations on the diet depending on the disease process.

The Kushi Institute is a strong proponent of the macrobiotic diet. The Institute is based in Massachusetts and teaches the macrobiotic diet and lifestyle. It recommends specific foods for the individual cancer patient. There have been numerous testimonials supporting the effectiveness of the macrobiotic diet in battling cancer. However, there have not been any controlled studies evaluating the Kushi Institutes' methods. The basic cost of the one-week program is $1,495, which includes the program, meals, and a room. Private counseling sessions are $225 each.

Here are some cautions for the cancer patient regarding the macrobiotic diet:

• The diet is very rigid and restrictive.

- Participants may lose a significant amount of weight, which can make standard cancer treatments harder to tolerate.
- Pregnant or nursing women should not use the macrobiotic diet.
- Children should not be placed on a macrobiotic diet. Children may not get the required nutrients to support proper growth and development.
- Avoid any promoters of dietary regimens who advise patients to stop conventional cancer treatments.
- If you are considering the macrobiotic diet, wait until completion of all conventional cancer treatments.

# PC-SPES Herbal Therapy for Prostate Cancer

Numerous herbal therapies are promoted for prostate health in the mass media. Some of these herbs include saw palmetto, PC-SPES, and lycopene. PC-SPES is a combination herbal preparation of eight different substances. It is not regulated by the FDA because it is considered a food supplement and not a medication. It contains chrysanthemum, isatis, licorice, *Ganoderma lucidum*, Panex-pseudo-ginseng, *Rabdosia rubescens,* saw palmetto, and Scutellaria. There is evidence that some of these compounds have similar activity to the female hormone estrogen. Licorice appears to stick to the estrogen receptor sites on cells. Ginseng induces the expression of gene products classically stimulated by estrogen.

An article published in the *New England Journal of Medicine* evaluated eight patients taking PC-SPES. It was found that the herbal combination caused the male sex hormone testosterone to decrease significantly in patients taking the supplement. All patients had a decrease in the PSA blood test that is used to screen and follow patients with prostate cancer. Also, patients experienced loss of libido, breast swelling, and breast tenderness. These same side effects are found when men are treated with medical doses of estrogen. Laboratory analysis of PC-SPES showed the herbal combination has potent activity similar to estrogen in yeast cells, mice, and humans.

It is clear that PC-SPES does have important effects on the prostate gland that are not totally understood to date. Clinical studies are ongoing, and more information is needed before PC-SPES can be recommended in the treatment of prostate cancer. Because many treatment decisions are based on the

PSA blood test and PC-SPES can cause a decrease in its level, physicians must know when patients are using this therapy. It is important that physicians ask patients about the use of PC-SPES and patients inform their healthcare provider about their use of the agent. No one wants the wrong treatment recommendation because the physician was not informed of all herbal therapies used by the patient.

# The Revici Method for the Treatment of Cancer

The Revici Method is an unconventional therapy for the treatment of cancer developed by Emanuel Revici. Revici believed that pathologic conditions were due to a chemical imbalance within the body that could be modified. The method is a blending of clinical observations, laboratory analyses, and chemotherapy. Basically, Revici would analyze the urine, blood, and body temperature and place patients in specific categories based on the "imbalance" that was discovered from these tests. The method was analyzed by a Clinical Appraisal Group consisting of a number of prominent physicians in 1965. Thirty-three patients treated by Revici were analyzed by the group of physicians. No instance of objective tumor regression was observed in any of the 33 case studies. In fact, 15 patients had autopsies after their deaths and there was no evidence of tumor alteration because of therapy.

Revici remained embattled with the New York State health authorities for years and had his medical license revoked in 1993 at the age of 96. Although Revici has died, his method remains highly touted in unconventional medical therapy books and on the Internet. In fact, a number of therapies that closely resemble the Revici method are now being touted by unconventional medical practitioners.

Biologic terrain assessment (BTA) is a therapy that is remarkably similar to the Revici Method and is promoted by some alternative medicine practitioners. It utilizes an analysis of the saliva, urine, and blood to isolate "imbalances." Herbal therapies are then prescribed to counteract these imbalances. In fact, practitioners of BTA claim that the herbal treatment can be directed to the organ containing the cancer to make it more effective. There is no objective evidence that BTA has any impact on cancer. There are no scientific studies evaluating its effectiveness. Some unconventional practitioners continue to claim that effectiveness has been proved based on case reports and testimonials, which are not valid scientific endpoints.

I do not recommend that patients use the Revici method or biologic terrain assessment. Any patient considering an unconventional medical therapy should discuss this option with his or her conventional medical physician. There can be important interactions with conventional cancer therapy or side effects of the therapy that you may not be aware.

*CancerTip*          **Saw Palmetto**

Saw palmetto is an herbal therapy whose active ingredient comes from the berries of the American dwarf palm. The plant thrives in the southeastern United States and it was originally used by the Seminole Indians as a medicinal. Saw palmetto is most commonly recommended for the treatment of benign prostatic hypertrophy (BPH), an enlarged prostate gland.

A number of clinical trials have been performed to evaluate the effectiveness of saw palmetto for control of the symptoms of BPH. A systematic review and analysis of all prospective trials including saw palmetto was reported in the *Journal of the American Medical Association*. Although the scientific literature is limited owing to variations in study designs, short duration of follow-up, and reporting of scientific outcomes, the evidence seems to favor some benefit to saw palmetto. Compared with the common prescription medication prescribed for BPH, saw palmetto showed similar improvement in urinary symptoms and urine flow with few side effects. The exact mechanism of action is unknown, although theories abound.

Saw palmetto is available in the form of tablets, capsules, teas, and berries. Although side effects are rare, they may include high blood pressure, abdominal pain, nausea, diarrhea, decreased sex drive, impotence, urinary retention, and headache. More scientific study is needed to fully evaluate the impact of saw palmetto on the (PSA) blood test. Until adequate data is available, it is prudent to discuss the use of this therapy with your physician, particularly in regard to the PSA blood test. The PSA level should be measured by your physician before starting therapy with saw palmetto to establish a baseline value. It must be emphasized that there is no evidence that saw palmetto is effective in the treatment of prostate cancer.

It should always be remembered that any herbal treatment can interact with conventional medications. This can cause alterations of blood levels of prescribed medications and alter the effectiveness of these medications. Also, the toxicities of conventional medications may be enhanced by an herbal therapy. Always take time to discuss the use of unconventional medications with your healthcare provider before starting any therapy.

*CancerTip* **Shark Cartilage**

Shark cartilage has gained increased popularity as an uncon-ventional cancer treatment and in prevention of cancer. Shark cartilage was initially promoted by William Lane in his book *Sharks Don't Get Cancer* and the follow-up book *Sharks Still Don't Get Cancer.* Unfortunately, sharks do get cancer. They develop melanoma, brain tumors, cancer of the blood system, and even cancer in the cartilage.

Shark cartilage is purported to contain angiogenesis in-hibitors, which prevent the formation of new blood vessels that tumors need to grow. A modest antiangiogenic effect has been seen in test tubes but not in humans at this point. Shark carti-lage is supplied in powder and capsule forms. It is taken orally and sometimes as an enema.

The news program *60 Minutes* gave shark cartilage therapy a huge boost a few years ago. The program reported a Cuban study of 29 patients with "terminal" cancer who were placed on shark cartilage. Most patients "felt better" several weeks after starting the shark cartilage. "Feeling better" is not a reliable endpoint in a scientific study. The National Cancer Institute (NCI) performed a review of the study and believed that the data was "incomplete and unimpressive." *60 Minutes* subsequently refused to broadcast the findings of the NCI.

A small study on shark cartilage was reported at the Ameri-can Society for Clinical Oncology (ASCO) in 1997. Patients with advanced cancer were given shark cartilage for 12 weeks. Of the 58 patients treated, there was not one complete response or partial response to shark cartilage. Only two patients had sig-nificant improvement in quality of life. A study reported at

ASCO in 1999 using shark cartilage for the treatment of brain tumors failed to show any significant tumor activity. There are some ongoing studies of shark cartilage at a number of institutions, but no positive trials have been published in the scientific literature.

Shark cartilage is relatively expensive. If it is taken as described by William Lane, the 16-week program cost is approximately $3,000. There are discount suppliers, but beware of using some sources. Some producers do not supply pure shark cartilage, and there may be additives and fillers.

There are some cautions for the cancer patient regarding shark cartilage:

- Children and pregnant women should not take shark cartilage because if the cartilage does work as an inhibitor of blood vessels, it could adversely affect growing children and the growing fetus.
- Those who have had recent surgery should not take shark cartilage because it can theoretically impair healing.
- Avoid using shark cartilage enemas if you are neutropenic (have a low white blood cell count). You can induce a life threatening infection.
- Some shark cartilage may contain additives, fillers, and contaminants.
- Shark cartilage can cause diarrhea, which can affect the patients ability to tolerate conventional cancer treatments.
- Shark cartilage has also been reported to cause hepatitis.

*CancerTip*          **Mind-Body Therapies**

Complementary medical techniques are gaining increased acceptance within the medical community. Some of the most helpful complementary techniques include the mind-body therapies. These include meditation, biofeedback, guided imagery, music therapy, art therapy, prayer, and hypnosis. Each of these methods may help the patient deal with anxiety, stress, and other subjective symptoms related to the diagnosis and treatment of cancer.

Meditation is a good technique that can be used to help with stress reduction. It is an easy technique to learn and can be done without the help of a therapist. It can be practiced in a variety of places including work, home, and in the hospital. Meditation originated in the Eastern religions and was used for calming and focusing the mind. It has been popularized in the United States through the introduction of transcendental meditation by Maharishi Mahesh Yogi in the 1960s. Deepak Chopra, who has been a strong supporter of meditation, has also helped spread its popularity.

There are many ways to practice meditation, and each individual develops his or her own style and preferences. Most recommend performing meditation once or twice a day for 10 to 20 minutes to reap the full benefits. Find a quiet spot where you will not be disturbed. Sit in a comfortable position with your back straight. Close your eyes so you are not affected by visual stimulation. Breathe naturally. Some use a mantra (phrase or word that you repeat to yourself to help distract your thoughts) such as "Om." Gradually relax all the muscles in your body from your feet up to your head. Your mind may wander, but use your mantra to help you continue to focus on your breathing and relaxation.

There are many wonderful books available to those interested in learning meditation. Browse through your local bookstore at the selection. One suggestion is a book entitled *Minding the Body, Mending the Mind*. Meditation is a wonderful complementary medical technique that is safe, relaxing, and best of all, free!

Guided Imagery is a technique that relies heavily on the power of suggestion to create relaxing mental images for the participants. It is particularly useful for relieving stress and relaxing the cancer patient. It is not a treatment for cancer, but some patients find that it helps them cope with the diagnosis and side effects of treatments more effectively.

The therapist will instruct the participants to visualize a specific image. Sometimes the participant is asked to visualize a mass of cancerous cells being attacked by the immune system, chemotherapy, or radiation therapy. Many patients use guided imagery audiotapes, which provide instruction on meditation exercises, guided relaxation, and visualization techniques. Some patients use these tapes while they are receiving their chemotherapy, radiation therapy, or traveling to their treatments.

The initial goal of guided imagery is total relaxation. Patients learn breathing exercises to help them attain an "inner calm." Patients then try to modify their anxiety or pain by imagining a pleasurable scene or situation.

Guided imagery may make a cancer patient feel better, but it does not cure cancer. Do not replace conventional medical treatments with guided imagery. It may be used effectively in some patients for relaxation and relief of anxiety. If you are interested in guided imagery, try starting with audiotapes specifically for cancer patients such as those produced by Petrea King or Belleruth Neparstak.

Emotional and physical stresses can be a heavy burden for the cancer patient. The diagnosis and treatment of cancer can make some patients feel as though they have lost control of their lives. Some patients turn to medications to help them deal with stress and anxiety. Others attend support group sessions or seek professional therapists. Still others take an approach such as biofeedback, which requires active participation and helps some patients feel that they have gained some control back in their lives.

Biofeedback manipulates the body's physiologic responses that are normally controlled by the autonomic nervous system. A biofeedback therapist, of which there are over 10,000 in the United States, can teach a patient how to control many of the body's involuntary functions. Some patients learn to control their heart rate, blood pressure, muscle tension, and emotions.

The therapist places monitoring electrodes on the body or scalp. The electrodes are then connected to a computer or polygraph. This will emit a noise or signal indicating the intensity or level of the process to be controlled. The patient is then instructed to concentrate on trying to influence the signal. Specific mental exercises will be performed under the direction of the therapist. The patient will visualize certain images that affect the mood. The patient may eventually learn which mental exercises change the signals. After a number of sessions (usually 8 to 10), the patient may be able to affect certain autonomic processes.

Biofeedback is a technique that can be useful in a wide variety of conditions. It is not used to cure cancer. The greatest benefit from biofeedback for the cancer patient is relaxation and reduction of stress. This can undoubtedly improve the quality of life for those who are successful. It allows the cancer patient to take an active role in his or her treatment. Biofeedback is noninvasive, inexpensive, and safe.

# MISCELLANEOUS TOPICS

*Cancer Tip*  # The Staging of Cancer

A number of cancer staging systems have evolved over the years. These systems have been developed to provide a way by which information on specific cancers can readily be communicated between health professionals. They are also used to assist in therapeutic decisions and to estimate prognosis for patients. The staging systems provide a mechanism for comparing similar groups of patients in the evaluation of therapeutic procedures.

Depending on the site of the cancer, a variety of tests may be recommended for a patient before the official stage is declared. These tests may include x-ray studies, computed tomography (CT) scans, magnetic resonance imaging (MRI) scans, bone scans, lymphangiograms, blood tests, and examinations under anesthesia, just to name a few. Each site of disease has specific tests that are required for proper staging to be performed. Staging of a patient without the use of surgical exploration is termed clinical staging. When surgery is performed as an exploratory procedure or resection of the cancer, this is called pathologic staging. It should always be noted whether the staging is clinical or pathologic.

The American Joint Committee on Cancer (AJCC) has developed the tumor-node-metastasis staging system (TNM) in an attempt to unify many of the various staging systems. This is identical to the classification of the Union Internationale Contre le Cancer (UICC). The classification is based on the premise that cancers of the same anatomic site and histology (what it looks like under a microscope) share similar patterns of growth and extension. The TNM system is defined individually for each site because of the different behavior of tumors at different sites. For most cancers, the TNM system is concerned with the anatomic extent of disease. There are some instances in which other factors such as the histologic grade of the tumor or age of the patient are incorporated into the staging system.

"T" stands for tumor. Small tumors are classified as T1, whereas locally advanced tumors with invasion into adjacent structures may be classified as T4. "N" stands for lymph nodes. Those tumors without lymph node involvement are classified as N0. Patients with positive lymph nodes have progressively higher values assigned depending on the extent of disease. "M" stands for metastases. Those patients without evidence of metastatic disease after complete staging work-up are classified as M0.

A patient with a small tumor, no lymph node involvement and no evidence of metastatic disease would be classified as T1N0M0 based on the TNM classification system. These classifications can then be grouped into stages.

Once a patient's disease is declared as a particular stage, that stage never changes. If a patient was diagnosed with an early stage cancer (stage I) but then develops metastatic disease after the completion of definitive treatment, the patient is considered to have stage I disease with metastases. This allows the medical community to compare the outcomes of particular treatments. If a patient's stage was changed with a recurrence or metastases, it would be too confusing to compare outcomes.

There are other staging systems for particular cancers that are commonly used. The Ann Arbor classification for Hodgkin's disease, the Federation Internationale de Gynecologie et d'Obstetrique (FIGO) for carcinomas of gynecologic sites, and the American Urologic Association (AUA) staging for prostate cancer are used frequently in adult cancers. There are a number of different staging systems in use for the pediatric cancers.

It is very important that patients are staged appropriately after the diagnosis of cancer. Patients should question their physicians about the staging work-up and consult with an oncologist that specializes in the treatment of their specific type of cancer.

# Beware of Media Hype: "A New Cancer Cure"

Beware of claims in the media of "a new cure for cancer." It is natural for the cancer patient to believe in media hype and accept claims of "cure" at face value. Many patients feel desperate and that they lack control of their lives. When respected news organizations announced that a combination of two research drugs (endostatin and angiostatin) could "cure cancer in 2 years," cancer patients throughout the world were given new hope. Unfortunately, as in previously reported "cures" for cancer, it may be many years before these drugs can be used in the general population. These drugs have been shown to cure tumors in mice, not humans. Many treatments have worked for various diseases in mice and have failed in human trials. These drugs have a long way to go before they can be approved in treatments of human cancers.

The media has a tendency to blow medical reports out of proportion and sensationalize new treatments. Over the past 15 years other treatments were labeled as "new cures for cancer," including monoclonal antibodies, interferon, interleukin-2 (IL-2), and tumor necrosis factor (TNF). Each treatment has found a limited role in the treatment of specific cancers but are in no way a cure for cancer on their own.

Cancer is not just a single disease. It is a conglomeration of over one hundred different diseases, with different cells and different genetic mutations. There is little chance that a single treatment will cure all cancers. Most cancers require multi-modality treatments with some combination of surgery, chemotherapy, or radiation therapy. Each of these modalities treats an individual cancer with specific techniques that may not be effective in other types of cancers. Cancer can also become resistant to a specific type of therapy, which requires the integration of other approaches in treatment.

The most effective way to eradicate cancer is to prevent its occurrence. Any individual can significantly reduce their risk of cancer by avoiding smoking, drinking alcohol with moderation, eating a low fat diet, and protecting oneself from overexposure to the sun. The second most effective treatment is early detection of cancer. Cancers are much more treatable when they are diagnosed at an early stage, so follow age-appropriate screening recommendations for specific cancers. Screening mammograms, gynecologic examinations, stool occult blood tests, colonoscopies, digital rectal examinations, and prostate specific antigen (PSA) blood tests have been proved to help detect cancer at an earlier stage. It is also important for the general population to learn self-screening techniques such as the breast self-examination, testicular self-examination, and skin self-examination.

Contrary to popular belief, there is not a big conspiracy by the medical establishment to prevent the public from gaining access to new treatments. Unfortunately, it takes many years to identify a new treatment, show that it is safe, prove that it works better than established treatments, and then produce enough of the treatment to make it widely available.

There are many new, exciting ways to treat cancer that are currently under investigation. The only way to identify the most promising new treatments is to test them in clinical research trials. If you have been diagnosed with cancer, ask your physician about any clinical research trials that you may be eligible to join. You may not only help yourself, but the many other patients who are diagnosed with cancer in the future.

Again, beware of media claims of a "new cure for cancer." These are exciting times in cancer research, but we still have a long way to go. Science is slowly unraveling the secrets of the many diseases known as cancer.

*CancerTip*          **Considering Hospice**

The word "hospice" may scare patients and family members when they hear the term for the first time. Hospice is generally recommended when a patient has less than 6 months to live. A referral from a doctor is required to be accepted into a hospice program. Patients must decide to give up on curative treatments for palliative supportive comfort care only. At first, it may be a shock for the patient to face his or her own mortality. Once patients realize the benefits of hospice, there is usually a great sense of relief.

Hospice provides support in the home at every level. Hospice workers and volunteers include nurses, physical therapists, social workers, nutritionists, chaplains, and home health aids. There are even transportation services. Almost all medical care is provided in the home environment. The overall goal of the hospice team is to enhance the quality of the remainder of the patients' life.

The hospice nurse becomes the eyes and ears of your physician. Instead of making trips to the physicians' office or hospital, most interactions take place over the telephone. The nurse keeps your doctor informed on your medical condition and medication needs. You may still visit with your doctor, but the goal is to provide most services in the home.

Although hospice is provided for patients who are dying of their disease, it can greatly enhance the quality of the patients' remaining life. Hospice also provides extensive assistance and support to the caregivers at home. This alleviates the fear many patients have of becoming a burden on the family. It also allows the patient to die with dignity in a comfortable environment.

When a patient develops end-stage cancer that is refractory to medical treatments, hospice may be recommended by your physician. The patient and family should ask about hospice care if medical treatment options have been exhausted and they are comfortable with comfort care. Hospice provides valuable services to the patient and family when they are needed the most.

*CancerTip*  **Radiation Therapy**

Radiation therapy is used in the treatment of a wide variety of cancers. It is also used to treat some benign conditions. Radiation oncologists are physicians who specialize in the treatment of malignant and benign diseases with radiation therapy. Radiation therapy works by attacking the genetic material located in the nucleus of a cell. Radiation does not instantly kill most cells. The cells die when they attempt the next cell division. This is why radiation therapy can continue to work for weeks or months after the treatment has been completed.

There are two ways to deliver radiation therapy: brachytherapy and external beam radiation therapy. Brachytherapy is the delivery of radiation by placing radioactive sources in the patient. These sources may be temporary or permanent. External beam radiation therapy is the use of gamma rays or x-rays that originate from an external source directed toward the patient. Most patients treated in radiation oncology centers receive external beam radiation therapy. A machine called a linear accelerators is used to generate high energy x-ray beams to treat patients. These are the most common machines used in radiation oncology centers. Some centers use cobalt machines that contain a strong radioactive source to produce gamma rays. Other specialized machines may be used in some facilities to treat skin cancers.

When patients are treated with external beam radiation therapy, there are a number of planning steps that must be taken before the first treatment is delivered. After a consultation with the radiation oncologist, special radiologic studies may be ordered to help plan the radiation treatments. Devices may need to be fabricated to keep the patient in the proper position during treatment. These may include masks, casts, molds, and special mouthpieces depending on the area of the body that requires treatment.

Next, a simulation is performed. This session usually takes approximately one hour. The simulator is a machine that looks like a linear accelerator except that it has a diagnostic x-ray unit attached. This allows the physician to plan accurately the radiation treatment fields based on the tumor position and anatomy of the patient. The radiation oncologist plans the size of the radiation field and the directions from which the patient will be treated. Once the radiation oncologist is satisfied with the field arrangement, small tattoos are placed on the skin to mark the treatment field. The tattoos look like small, blue freckles. These help ensure that the radiation fields are set up properly each day of treatment. Blocks will be fabricated based on the simulation x-rays to shield normal structures and minimize side effects. The blocks will take a day or two to create because they are custom made for each patient.

After the treatment plan is completed and blocks are finished, the patient returns for a set-up session. The set up takes approximately 30 minutes. During this time, the radiation oncologist confirms the field arrangements and checks the blocks for proper alignment based on the x-rays taken at the time of simulation. Adjustments are made accordingly. If everything lines up correctly, treatments may start as directed by the radiation oncologist.

The patient should plan on spending approximately 30 minutes in the radiation department each day. The patient will be in the treatment room for 10 to 15 minutes. Most of the time is spent placing the patient in the correct position. The radiation machine is "on" for only 1 to 2 minutes. There is no sensation involved when the machine is delivering the radiation. The patient is not radioactive after treatment with external beam radiation therapy.

Side effects of radiation therapy are related to the area of the body being treated, dose of radiation delivered each day, and total dose of radiation given over a treatment course. The radiation oncologist discusses the side effects associated with a particular treatment before starting therapy. Radiation therapy may last from 1 day to 3 weeks for palliative treatments and approximately several weeks for definitive (curative) treatments. The length of treatment is determined on an individual basis. Treatments are typically given 5 days a week, Monday through Friday. Treatments are not usually given over the weekend except for emergencies.

Emergencies such as spinal cord compression, superior vena cava syndrome, and brain metastases may require modifications to the above-mentioned procedures. It may be important to start treatment immediately on these patients before the cancer causes catastrophic complications. In these situations, the radiation oncologist plans the radiation treatment so it can start without delay.

# Herceptin and Breast Cancer

Herceptin is a monoclonal antibody that was recently approved by the Food and Drug Administration (FDA) for the treatment of a special type of metastatic breast cancer. It is directed at those breast cancers that overexpress a specific protein on the surface of the cancer cell. This protein is called HER-2/nue (pronounced "her two new"). It is found to be overexpressed in about 30% of breast cancers. Those cancers that overexpress HER-2/nue may be more aggressive than those that do not.

Recent studies have shown Herceptin to be of benefit to patients with metastatic breast cancer who have overexpression of HER-2/nue. One study of metastatic breast cancer patients receiving doxorubicin-cyclophosphamide (AC) or paclitaxel chemotherapy randomized patients to receive Herceptin along with the other drugs or no additional therapy. There were significant improvements in time to disease progression and response rates in the group that received Herceptin in addition to the other chemotherapy.

Acute side effects of Herceptin included fever and chills. There has also been an increased incidence of gastrointestinal problems such as diarrhea when Herceptin is given in combination with chemotherapy. One major side effect of concern is an increased risk of cardiac toxicity when Herceptin is combined with anthracycline-based chemotherapy. A study showed that 27% percent of patients experienced cardiac toxicity compared with only 7% of those taking anthracycline alone and 11% of those taking the paclitaxel and Herceptin combination. Because this is a new treatment, more side effects may become evident as increased numbers of patients use the treatment.

Herceptin is being evaluated as a treatment for other solid tumors with overexpression of HER-2/nue. Herceptin is approved only for the treatment of certain types of breast cancer, but there are a number of studies evaluating other cancers. Patients who are interested in this new treatment should ask their physician if they are eligible to participate in the ongoing clinical trials.

*Cancertip*  # Photodynamic Therapy

Photodynamic therapy (PDT) is a new light-based cancer treatment that is under investigation for a variety of malignancies. It is currently approved by the FDA for the treatment of esophageal cancer and lung cancer that is obstructing an airway. It is being investigated for a variety of other clinical situations. There are a number of exciting research trials ongoing at the Hospital of the University of Pennsylvania. These include PDT for the treatment of mesothelioma, locally advanced lung cancer with a malignant pleural effusion, recurrent pleural effusions from a variety of cancers, and cancers that have seeded the abdominal cavity, including carcinomas, sarcomas, and ovarian cancers. There are a number of protocols being developed for other sites in the body. You can search the UPCC protocol finder for current photodynamic therapy studies available at the Hospital of the University of Pennsylvania on the Internet (http://www.oncolink.upenn.edu/clinical_trials/protocols.html).

How does photodynamic therapy work? A medication that sensitizes the individual to light is given 1 to 7 days before the photodynamic therapy procedure. The only FDA-approved medication is called porfimer sodium (Photofrin). This agent is given by an intravenous infusion over about 15 minutes. There are some indications that tumor cells pick up the drug more readily than normal cells. The drug is not active against the tumor cells by itself. It must be activated by a specific wavelength of light to kill cancer cells. At this point, the patient is sensitive to light and must take appropriate precautions.

The following is a general outline of what happens next. Your physician will give you specific details depending on the site being treated. On the specified day, the patient returns and is taken to the operating room for the PDT treatment. A surgical resection of any visible tumor will be performed prior to the PDT treatment. To proceed with the photodynamic therapy, the patient must only have minimal residual disease after a surgical resection. If the surgeon is unable to remove the tumor so only a thin layer of cells remains (less than 5 mm), the procedure is not performed. The laser light that is used in the treatment can only penetrate about 5 mm into tissue. If there is disease thicker than this, the treatment will be ineffective.

A laser is used in the surgical cavity to activate the drug and kill remaining cancer cells. The drug is now active only in the areas exposed to the laser. Once all of the areas at risk have received the specified dose of light, the treatment is completed. This complete procedure is performed while the patient is under general anesthesia. Once the photodynamic therapy is complete, the surgeon closes the wound and the surgery is finished. Photodynamic therapy typically adds 1 to 2 hours to the operative time.

Side effects of treatment are dependent on the area of the body to be treated and extent of surgical resection. The treating physician addresses these site-specific side effects at the time of consultation. All patients who receive the photosensitizing drug will become sensitive to light. Light sensitization occurs once the drug is infused. Depending on the medication used, the patient may be sensitive to light for approximately 4 to 6 weeks. Specific instructions are given by the treating physician on how to avoid direct sunlight. Sun exposure may cause a blistering burn within a minute. It is imperative the patient follow the directions on light exposure.

*CancerTip*  **Viatical Settlements**

A viatical settlement is the purchase of a life insurance policy from a terminally ill patient in exchange for a cash percentage of the policies worth. Patients can sell all or part of their life insurance policy for immediate cash. Viatical settlements are not for everyone, but they are an important option for those that need money to pay bills, cover expensive home care, or replace income from lost employment. Approximately 31% of families become impoverished while managing the illness of a loved one with terminal disease. Viatical settlements are one option to avoid such a situation.

How do viatical settlements work? The seller of an insurance policy names the purchaser as beneficiary. A viatical company is the purchaser of the policy. In exchange, the seller receives a lump sum payment at the time of the sale. The amount paid for an applicant's policy is determined by the prevailing interest rates, premium obligations, projected life expectancy, and face value of the policy. The seller usually receives between 45% to 60% of the face value of the policy. The purchaser of the policy becomes responsible for all future premium payments, regardless of how long the seller lives. There are no restrictions on how the funds can be used. The entire process usually takes about 1 month. Most insurance policies qualify for settlements.

Owing to the Health Insurance Portability and Accountability Act, individuals with chronic or life-threatening illnesses may be able to receive viatical settlement proceeds free from any federal income tax. A viatical settlement can be structured so that it does not affect needs-based entitlements such as those from Social Security and Disability Insurance.

In the United States, viatical companies are required to obtain a license in most states. Make sure that the company is legitimate. Check with your state Consumer Affairs Office or Insurance Commissioner to determine whether there have been any complaints lodged against the company.

*CancerTip*

# Finding the Right Cancer Book

You or a family member has been diagnosed with cancer. You are starving for good information about cancer. So, you decide to go to the bookstore or shop online for "THE BOOK." The problem is you find there are a couple of shelves filled with books on the topic of cancer or pages of book titles on the Internet. The question then arises, "How Do I Pick the Right Book?" It can be confusing with hundreds of books about cancer for sale. Many of them sound good according to the cover, but you should always wonder if they give reliable information.

First of all, there is probably no book out there that can be considered "THE BOOK" for everyone. Each person is looking for something different in a book. Some want basic facts, some want encouragement, some want to find a way of gaining control over their lives after a diagnosis of cancer.

Before looking for a book, ask your physician if he or she recommends any particular resources. Your physician has undoubtedly looked at a number of references and can recommend some reliable reading material. Support groups also are good places to learn about books.

OncoLink has a large and reliable book review section. All books are reviewed by physicians and other expert healthcare professionals. Only books that fulfill our strict criteria for excellence are recommended to our users. The book review section is divided by topic for easy use. Unfortunately, there are some books that give false or misleading information, and a section has been created to warn OncoLink users about these kinds of books.

There are no books that address every type of cancer completely and effectively. Most people should buy two types of cancer books to get most of the information they will need. The first type of book that everyone should have is a general cancer reference book. These books offer an overview of cancer diagnosis and the variety of general treatments available. They explain the three major treatments for cancer including chemotherapy, surgery, and radiation therapy. They also discuss supportive care and quality of life issues. Good overviews are easy to read, define medical jargon, and leave the reader feeling that he or she understands the basic terms. It should also contain a reference list including Internet resources, organizations and support groups, and recommended books.

Next, you should look for a book that specifically addresses the type of cancer you are interested in learning the most about. This book should detail the diagnosis, staging, treatment, and follow-up for this particular cancer. It should detail all of the treatment options and side effects of therapy.

Starting with these two types of books will give you a good start on understanding the diagnosis and treatment of a cancer. There may be other books that interest you but these first two types of books will give you a strong foundation for more specific reading.

| SECTION VIII | # INTERNET GUIDE TO USEFUL CANCER INFORMATION |
|---|---|

|              | **Use of the Internet to** |
| *CancerTip*  | **Obtain Cancer-Related** |
|              | **Information** |

There has been an explosion in the use of the Internet to gather cancer-related information. The Internet provides a powerful tool for patients and healthcare providers to gather new and useful information. A frequent question from Internet users is "how do I know what is a good website?" This simple question requires a more complex answer.

The editorial staff at OncoLink has reviewed thousands of cancer-related websites. We are constantly evaluating new sites and reevaluating older ones. A number of parameters have been developed to grade specific sites. We have given the best sites on the Internet "OncoLink Editors Choice Awards." The following are the parameters that should be used in the evaluation of a medical website.

1. Accuracy—Information should be correct and truthful. The author's name and date of posting should be included with each document. References should be included when appropriate.
2. Updated Content—Content on an Internet site should be updated regularly. This gives an indication of how well the site is managed. Sites that are not updated for months at a time should be avoided. Remember that although some basic things do not change much, there is always new medical information that can be added to a website.
3. Editorial Staff—Make sure the editorial staff is listed and has proper credentials to give medical advice. There are many sites that give medical information without proper medical training. The site should also provide addresses of the editor's or e-mail contact information. They should be available to respond to questions about the Internet site.

4. Reputation—Those sites run by reputable institutions are more likely to provide responsible and accurate information.

5. Sales—A number of sites sell products over the Internet. Many of these items are useful in particular circumstances. However, beware of sites that are created only to sell a product. These sites may contain biased and misleading information.

6. Organization—Make sure the site is easy to use and has a good search engine.

7. Awards—Sites that have received numerous awards from reputable sources most likely are reliable. Most editors will post a list of the awards that have been bestowed on the website.

8. Conflicts of Interest—any conflicts of interest should be disclosed to the users.

The following is a list of websites that have been carefully reviewed using the parameters listed above. These sites are deemed the highest of quality in their particular category.

*CancerTip*

# General Cancer Information Sites

**OncoLink** (http://www.oncolink.upenn.edu)—The University of Pennsylvania Cancer Center's Internet resource. Recognized as the top Internet health information site by the GII Award, OncoLink provides reliable and complete information for cancer patients, families, and healthcare providers and physicians. The site provides comprehensive cancer information, tips for cancer patients, book reviews, online journals, video lectures, and a multitude of other topics supported by cancer experts.

**The American Cancer Society** (http://www.cancer.org/)—The American Cancer Society was founded in 1913 and is devoted to disseminating knowledge concerning the symptoms, treatment, and prevention of cancer; to investigate conditions under which cancer is found; and to compile statistics in regard thereto. The American Cancer Society home page contains a plethora of information on line. This ranges from how to get a ride to treatment to information about marriage counseling. A listing of the numerous chartered divisions is provided. This is an outstanding resource.

**National Cancer Institute: Physician's Data Query (PDQ) Statements** (http://www.oncolink.upenn.edu/pdq/)—Physician's Data Query (PDQ) is the National Cancer Institute's (NCI) most up-to-date source of cancer information. It has been distributed since 1984 and is now available in multiple forms including fax, e-mail, conventional mail, and the World Wide Web. Both English and Spanish versions are maintained. The information is edited by several boards of medical professionals representing virtually all cancer subspecialties. Updates are provided monthly and are directed both at healthcare professionals and at the public. This is an outstanding resource.

*CancerTip*  # Disease-Specific Sites

**International Myeloma Foundation** (http://myeloma.org/imf.html)—The International Myeloma Foundation is a non profit organization that is dedicated to improving the quality of life for multiple myeloma patients and ultimately to preventing and curing myeloma. Their website contains a wealth of information for patients and healthcare providers about this disease. Information is updated frequently. The IMF Newsletter "Myeloma Today" is available in a web version. This is an outstanding resource for patients, families, and others interested in multiple myeloma.

**The Body** (http://www.thebody.com/index.shtml)—The comprehensive acquired immunodeficiency syndrome (AIDS) and human immunodeficiency (HIV) information resource. The Body's mission is to use the Web to lower barriers between patients and clinicians, demystify HIV/AIDS and its treatment, improve patients' quality of life, and foster community through human connection.

**Testicular Cancer Resource Center** (http://www.acor.org/TCRC/)—This outstanding, comprehensive site maintained by testicular cancer survivors contains valuable information about this cancer including self-examination, posttreatment sexuality, testicular implants, and personal experiences.

**Lymphoma Research Foundation of America** (http://www.lymphoma.org)—This website was founded in 1991 by Ellen Glesby Cohen after she was diagnosed with non-Hodgkin's lymphoma. It was the first organization targeted specifically at funding lymphoma research on a national basis. Its goal is to promote and support high-quality research that will produce better treatments and ultimately result in a cure for the disease.

**American Brain Tumor Association** (http://www.abta.org/) (ABTA)—This website was founded in 1973 by two families who lost children to brain tumors. They vowed to find answers through research. Today, ABTA is a global organization making major strides by funding brain tumor research and providing the information patients need to make educated decisions about their health care.

**National Cervical Cancer Coalition** (http://www.nccc-on-line.org/)—This is an excellent website from a grass roots organization whose mission is to enhance awareness of the traditional Pap smear, new technologies and reimbursement issues facing cervical cancer screening. This effort is directed toward legislators to communicate the continued importance and success of cervical cancer screening as a national communicable disease and cancer screening test to lower cervical cancer rates, with emphasis on access to quality testing for all women.

**Childhood Leukemia Center** (http://www.patientcenters. com/leukemia/)—This center has been created especially for parents and others caring for a child with leukemia or other cancer. The material in this center has been excerpted or adapted from the book entitled *Childhood Leukemia: A Guide for Families, Friends, and Caregivers* by Nancy Keene.

**The Brain Tumor Society** (http://www.tbts.org/)—Home page of organization dedicated to the cure of brain tumors "through research, education and support." The page includes high-quality FAQs, information concerning grant support, support group information, and numerous internal and external links of interest to patients and professionals. This is an outstanding resource!

*CancerTip*

# Comprehensive and Reference Sites

The National Library of Medicine's **MEDLINEplus** (http://www.nlm.nih.gov/medlineplus/)—These pages are designed to direct consumers to resources containing information that will help patients research their health questions.

**NCBI PubMed: Literature Searches** (http://www4.ncbi.nlm.nih.gov/PubMed/)—PubMed is an experimental service of the National Center for Biotechnology Information (NCBI) at the National Library of Medicine (NLM), developed in conjunction with publishers of biomedical literature as a search tool for accessing literature citations and linking to their full-text versions at publishers' websites. PubMed searches the 8 million citations in MEDLINE supplemented by pre-Medline citations that do not yet have MeSH index terms and by citations supplied electronically by publishers. There is no charge for its use, and no registration is required.

**Women's Cancer Network (WCN)** (http://www.wcn.org/)—This outstanding site developed by the Gynecologic Cancer Foundation keeps women informed and enables them to be their own health advocates. The WCN mission is to assist women who have developed cancer, as well as their families, to understand more about the disease, learn about treatment options, and gain access to new or experimental therapies. The WCN Referral Guide enables women to find appropriate cancer treatment specialists in their area. WCN News provides a daily newsfeed from Reuters Health Information, with articles selected by women's cancer experts. The WCN serves to educate women in ways to prevent the development of cancer. WCN's confidential risk-assessment questionnaire is designed to give women a personalized understanding of their individual risks of developing breast, ovarian, cervical, or endometrial cancer.

**American Institute for Cancer Research Online** (http://www.aicr.org)—The American Institute for Cancer Research is the leading national charity in the field of diet, nutrition, and cancer prevention. The information you will find here could help you begin to reduce cancer risk for you and your family.

**Understanding Gene Testing: A booklet from the Department of Health and Human Services NIH and NCI** (http://www.accessexcellence.org/AE/AEPC/NIH/index.html) —This booklet is an illustrated, well written, and easy to read guide that explains basic genetics. The role, benefits, limitations, and risks of genetic testing for cancer are explored.

*CancerTip*

# Alternative Treatments Sites

The University of Texas Center for Alternative Medicine Research (UT-CAM) (http://www.sph.uth.tmc.edu/utcam/)—UT-CAM is dedicated to investigating the effectiveness of alternative and complementary therapies used for cancer prevention and control. The Center's mission is to facilitate the scientific evaluations of biopharmacologic and herbal therapies as well as innovative approaches; establish a national network of alternative medicine practitioners, conventional practitioners, and researchers; and support the use of critical evaluation skills among alternative medicine practitioners and researchers.

**Hotwired: HotSeat: If it Ducks Like a Quack** (http://www.hotwired.com/packet/hotseat/97/21/index4a.html)—an outstanding RealAudio based interview with John H. Renner and Wiliam Silberg of the *Journal of the American Medical Association (JAMA)*. They discuss many issues surrounding medical misinformation on the Internet and credibility of websites providing medical information. There is a related editorial in *JAMA* 1997;277:1244–1245.

**Quackwatch: A special message to cancer patients seeking alternative treatments** (http://www.quackwatch.com/00AboutQuackwatch/Altseek.html)—This is an Internet site that attempts to identify misinformation and false claims regarding treatment techniques and medications. This is a website that goes on the offensive against those who disseminate misinformation or advocate unproved therapy. It takes a "no nonsense" approach, which includes attacks on those who spread the misinformation. It consists of a good overview of alternative cancer treatments, along with references to sources of reliable information for cancer patients. The page is updated regularly. It continues to post many comments both supportive and critical of itself.

*CancerTip*  **Home Care Sites**

**American College of Physicians: Home Care Guide for Advanced Cancer** (http://www.acponline.org/public/h_care/)—This adjunct to the *American College of Physicians Home Care Guide for Cancer* addresses end-of-life issues that concern cancer patients, their families, and friends. The primary goal is to help plan near the end of life, and to maximize the patient's quality of life during this difficult time. This is a comprehensive and extremely well constructed publication that addresses everything from pain control to grieving, to helping younger people cope with death. For those concerned, it is required reading.

*CancerTip*          **Supportive Care Sites**

**PainLink** (http://www.edc.org/PainLink/)—An initiative of the Education Development Center, Inc. supported by The Mayday Fund. This site ". . . enables pain clinicians and other medical professionals at sites around the country to communicate with each other in an effort to improve patient care and reduce suffering."

**NPR: End of Life: Exploring Death in America** (http://www.npr.org/programs/death/)—This outstanding site from National Public Radio eloquently deals with the most difficult subject we all must face—our own death and the death of those who are close to us. Included are transcripts from their week-long report on death along with references and a roundtable discussion in Real Audio format. Poetry, artwork, references and suggested reading round out this comprehensive site.

*CancerTip*        **Coping Sites**

**NCI/NIH: Taking Time: Support for People With Cancer and the People Who Care About Them** (http://www.cancernet.nci.nih.gov/taking_time/timeintro.html)—This guide is dedicated to the many people with cancer and their family members. It provides many insights into the special problems people with cancer face and the ways in which they have found the courage to cope with them. Who should you tell about your cancer? What about changing doctors? What about sex and body image? These topics and more are addressed with caring and insight.

**Talking With Your Child About Cancer** (http://www.cancernet.nci.nih.gov/talking_to_kids/)—Learning that a child has cancer is perhaps the hardest news a parent ever has to face. The NCI/NIH offers this brochure, which includes age-appropriate advice for dealing with this difficult topic.

**NCI: Young People With Cancer, A Handbook for Parents** (http://www.cancernet.nci.nih.gov/young_people/yngconts.html)—This is an outstanding guide for parents of children living with cancer from the NCI.

**Smoking Cessation Sites**

**ACS: Smokeout** (http://www2.cancer.org/gas/)—This is an outstanding site by the American Cancer Society to celebrate the Smokeout campaign. The focus is to prevent students from starting smoking and to encourage them to stop if they have already become addicted. This site contains a wealth of information about smoking-related issues. Be sure to take part in the Smokeout petition and take the Smokeout pledge that reminds us that ". . . more people die every year from smoking-related diseases than from AIDS, alcohol, car accidents, fires, drugs, murders, and suicides combined."

**The QuitNet** (http://www.quitnet.org/)—This comprehensive, well-designed site from the Massachusetts Tobacco Control Program entitled *Join Together Online* focuses on tobacco control and smoking cessation. This is one of the best sites that we have seen to help people end their nicotine addiction.

**Dale Pray: Quit Smoking Cigarettes** (http://www.megalink.net/~dale/quitcigs.html)—This page highlight's Dale's 27-year battle with tobacco addiction, and contains numerous links to quitting smoking resources. Of particular interest is the "Smokers Suck Because . . ." portion of the resource. This page has been selected for being the best antismoking page I have seen.

# CANCER WORKBOOK

## MEDICATION LIST

It is very important for cancer patients to keep a list of all medications they are currently taking. The number of pills can be staggering at times, and it is very easy for patients to become confused. It is important to carry the list at all times so patients can show the doctors and nurses what medications are being taken. Cancer patients may be under the care of a number of different physicians and all of the doctors may not know what others have prescribed. Significant interactions can occur with some medicines that your doctor needs to consider before prescribing any new medication.

If a patient ever goes to the emergency room, a list of current medications is extremely helpful to the emergency room staff. Treatment can be instituted promptly if the doctors know all of the current medications the patient is taking. It is not real helpful to say "I'm taking a big blue pill." There are thousands of medications available that can have serious interactions. Keeping a list makes everyone's life easier.

It is important to list the name of each medication, the dose in milligrams, and the frequency that the medication is prescribed. The doctor who prescribed the medication and the date started should also be listed. The following is a sample list that can be copied and kept in a purse or wallet once the blanks have been filled:

## PRESCRIPTION MEDICATIONS

| Name of Medicine | Dose (mg) | Frequency Taking | Physician who Prescribed | Date Started | Reason for Medicine |
|---|---|---|---|---|---|
| | | | | | |
| | | | | | |
| | | | | | |
| | | | | | |
| | | | | | |
| | | | | | |
| | | | | | |
| | | | | | |
| | | | | | |
| | | | | | |

## VITAMINS, HERBS, AND UNCONVENTIONAL MEDICAL TREATMENTS UTILIZED

There has been a dramatic increase in interest surrounding the use of herbs, vitamins, and unconventional medical treatments by the public. Most patients do not tell their physicians about the use of these treatments. Many times the patient does not consider these medicines and neglects to inform their physician about utilization of these substances. Sometimes the patient feels uncomfortable discussing these treatments with their doctor. It is important to have an open dialogue with the physicians responsible for your care. Many of these therapies can have interactions with conventional medications. They may also cause side effects that could wrongly be attributed to either the disease process or conventional treatments. For these reasons, your healthcare provider should be notified about these treatments.

Always keep a list of all vitamin supplements and herbs that are being taken. Over-the-counter medications are important to list also. Your doctor must know EVERYTHING that you are taking to treat you appropriately. Use the following chart to document any vitamins, herbs, or other unconventional treatments that are being utilized:

## VITAMINS, HERBS, AND UNCONVENTIONAL MEDICAL TREATMENTS

| Name of Vitamin, Herb, etc. | Dose (mg) | Frequency Utilized | Date Started | Reason for Treatment |
|---|---|---|---|---|
|  |  |  |  |  |
|  |  |  |  |  |
|  |  |  |  |  |
|  |  |  |  |  |
|  |  |  |  |  |
|  |  |  |  |  |
|  |  |  |  |  |
|  |  |  |  |  |
|  |  |  |  |  |
|  |  |  |  |  |

# MEDICAL HISTORY

It is important for your physician to know about any other medical problems that you have experienced. Providing this information helps your physician treat you in an appropriate manner. It also allows them to better discuss the side effects of treatment. List all medical problems, both current and resolved:

| Medical Problem | Date of Diagnosis | Treatment Received | Physician Responsible |
|---|---|---|---|
| | | | |
| | | | |
| | | | |
| | | | |
| | | | |
| | | | |
| | | | |

## PAST SURGICAL PROCEDURES

List any surgical procedures that you have experienced, no matter how long ago. Also, note the reason for each surgery. Do not forget to list the following procedures if they have been performed: tonsillectomy, gall bladder removal, appendectomy, and removal of skin cancers. These all count as surgery. Note any complications that you have experienced from the surgery.

| Surgery | Reason for Surgery | Date of Surgery | Surgeon | Complications |
|---|---|---|---|---|
| | | | | |
| | | | | |
| | | | | |
| | | | | |
| | | | | |

## PAST HOSPITALIZATIONS

Make a list of any previous hospital admissions. Make sure the date, name of hospital, and reason for hospitalization is included. Taking time to think about any hospitalizations will help you identify past medical issues. Use the following chart to help organize this important information.

| Date | Reason for Hospitalization | Name of Hospital | Responsible Physician |
|---|---|---|---|
| | | | |
| | | | |
| | | | |
| | | | |
| | | | |
| | | | |

# FAMILY HISTORY OF CANCER

Your physician will ask you about any other family members that have developed cancer. There are a number of cancers that have genetic links. In particular, take time to think about parents, grandparents, and siblings that may have experienced a diagnosis of cancer. Also, note the approximate age at which these family members were diagnosed with cancer. This information can help your physician determine if genetic testing or counseling should be performed.

| Name of Family Member | Relationship | Type of Cancer | Age of Diagnosis |
|---|---|---|---|
| | | | |
| | | | |
| | | | |
| | | | |
| | | | |

## CHEMOTHERAPY HISTORY

Many patients treated for cancer receive chemotherapy during some part of their treatment course. Chemotherapy is typically given in "cycles." Each cycle typically lasts three to four weeks. Patients may receive a number of different chemotherapy agents in combination or at different times during their treatment. It is important that all physicians involved in the patient's care are aware of the various agents that are utilized. There can be important side effects, interactions with medications, and interactions with radiation therapy for which physicians will be on the alert. Keep a record of the names of chemotherapy drugs, number of cycles, and the date of each cycle. The following chart will help organize this important information:

| Names of Chemotherapy | Date Cycle Started | Cycle Number | Medical Oncologist | Side Effects Noted |
|---|---|---|---|---|
| | | | | |
| | | | | |
| | | | | |
| | | | | |

## PHYSICIAN LIST

It is important for cancer patients to keep a list of all physicians involved in their medical care. Since most patients are treated with combined modality therapy for cancer, there may be multiple healthcare professionals involved in the care of the patient. Keeping a current list of physicians allows the patient to reference their physicians quickly. It is also important for all of your physicians to know who else is involved in your medical care. Notes updating your condition then can be sent to other physicians if you provide the names and addresses of everyone. This allows for care to flow smoothly since all of your physicians are updated regularly on your progress through treatment and follow up. It is important to keep the name, telephone number, fax number, address, and name of a nurse contact or secretary for each physician's office. The following chart can serve as an important guide. This list can be copied and handed to each of your physicians to place with your records.

**PHYSICIANS**

| Physician Name | Address | Phone/Fax Numbers | Specialty | Nurse Name | Secretary Name |
|---|---|---|---|---|---|
| | | | | | |
| | | | | | |
| | | | | | |
| | | | | | |
| | | | | | |
| | | | | | |
| | | | | | |
| | | | | | |
| | | | | | |
| | | | | | |

## RADIOLOGY STUDIES LIST

Most cancer patients will have numerous radiologic studies performed during the work-up and follow-up of a specific cancer. These studies may include x-rays, CT scans, MRI scans, ultrasound studies, and bone scans, just to name a few. It is important to keep a list of all studies that have been performed. Many of these studies may be performed at different facilities and it is difficult for consulting physicians to know every study that has been done. It is important for the patient to provide a list of the tests completed and location where the study was performed. This helps each of your physicians to obtain the results of these procedures. Always follow-up on the results of each of your tests with the physician who ordered the study. Do not just assume the results are "OK" if you do not hear anything. Use the following chart to help keep track of each study that has been performed:

RADIOLOGY STUDIES

| Name of Procedure | Date Completed | Location of Study | Phone Number | Physician Ordering Study | Discussed Results (Yes/No) |
|---|---|---|---|---|---|
| | | | | | |
| | | | | | |
| | | | | | |
| | | | | | |
| | | | | | |
| | | | | | |
| | | | | | |
| | | | | | |
| | | | | | |
| | | | | | |

## RADIATION THERAPY HISTORY

Radiation therapy is utilized in the treatment of a significant number of cancer patients. Radiation can be delivered for either curative or palliative reasons. The amount of radiation therapy delivered is limited due to the normal tissue tolerance. It is important that your radiation oncologist is aware of any radiation that may have been delivered in the past. Patients should keep a record of when they are treated, location on the body treated, total dose delivered, and the name of the radiation oncologist responsible for delivering the treatments. Your physicians will be able to obtain more summaries that are detailed if required. Use the following chart to register any treatments with radiation therapy:

| Dates of Radiation | Body Part Treated | Total Dose | Radiation Oncologist | Address | Phone Number |
|---|---|---|---|---|---|
|  |  |  |  |  |  |
|  |  |  |  |  |  |
|  |  |  |  |  |  |
|  |  |  |  |  |  |

# UPCOMING APPOINTMENTS

Most patients are overwhelmed at the number of appointments that are scheduled for consultations, treatment, and follow-up of their cancer. It is difficult for anyone to keep all of these dates and times straight in their head. Keeping an appointment book is an easy way to make sure that you do not miss any of your scheduled physicians visits or tests. Make sure to add your next visit to the appointment book before leaving your physician's office.

| Date | Time | Doctor's Name | Address | Phone Number |
|------|------|---------------|---------|--------------|
|      |      |               |         |              |
|      |      |               |         |              |
|      |      |               |         |              |
|      |      |               |         |              |
|      |      |               |         |              |
|      |      |               |         |              |

# SUBJECT INDEX